Recent and Related Titles in Bioethics

Joseph S. Alper, Catherine Ard, Adrienne Asch, Jon Beckwith, Peter Conrad, and Lisa N. Geller, eds. *The Double-Edged Helix: Social Implications of Genetics in a Diverse Society*

Mark P. Aulisio, Robert M. Arnold, and Stuart J. Youngner, eds. *Ethics Consultation: From Theory to Practice*

Nancy Berlinger. *After Harm: Medical Error and the Ethics of Forgiveness*

Daniel Callahan and Angela A. Wasunna. *Medicine and the Market: Equity v. Choice*

Audrey R. Chapman and Mark S. Frankel, eds. *Designing Our Descendants: The Promises and Perils of Genetic Modifications*

Grant R. Gillett. *Bioethics in the Clinic: Hippocratic Reflections*

John D. Lantos. *The Lazarus Case: Life-and-Death Issues in Neonatal Intensive Care*

Carol Levine and Thomas H. Murray, eds. *The Cultures of Caregiving: Conflict and Common Ground among Families, Health Professionals, and Policy Makers*

John P. Lizza. *Persons, Humanity, and the Definition of Death*

Erik Parens, ed. *Surgically Shaping Children: Technology, Ethics, and the Pursuit of Normality*

Mark A. Rothstein, Thomas H. Murray, Gregory E. Kaebnick, and Mary Anderlik Majumder, eds. *Genetic Ties and the Family: The Impact of Paternity Testing on Parents and Children*

Thomas H. Murray, Consulting Editor in Bioethics

Neonatal Bioethics

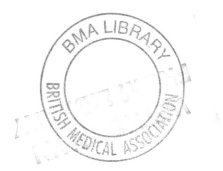

Neonatal Bioethics

The Moral Challenges of Medical Innovation

JOHN D. LANTOS, M.D.
Professor of Pediatrics and Medicine, and
Chief, Section of General Pediatrics
Department of Pediatrics
University of Chicago
Chicago, Illinois

and

WILLIAM L. MEADOW, M.D., Ph.D.
Professor of Pediatrics and Medicine
Co-Chief, Section of Neonatology
Department of Pediatrics
University of Chicago
Chicago, Illinois

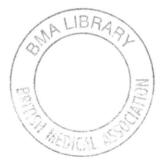

The Johns Hopkins University Press

Baltimore

2   4   6   8   9   7   5   3   1

The Johns Hopkins University Press
2715 North Charles Street
Baltimore, Maryland 21218-4363
www.press.jhu.edu

Library of Congress Cataloging-in-Publication Data
Lantos, John D.
Neonatal bioethics : the moral challenges of medical innovation /
John D. Lantos and William L. Meadow.
p. cm.
Includes bibliographical references and index.
ISBN 0-8018-8344-X (hardcover : alk. paper)
1. Neonatal intensive care—Moral and ethical aspects—United States.
2. Neonatology—Moral and ethical aspects—United States.
3. Neonatology—United States—History.
[DNLM: 1. Intensive Care Units, Neonatal—ethics—United States—Case Reports.
2. History, 20th Century—United States—Case Reports. 3. Intensive Care Units,
Neonatal—trends—United States—Case Reports. 4. Intensive Care, Neonatal—
ethics—United States—Case Reports. 5. Intensive Care, Neonatal—history—
United States—Case Reports. 6. Intensive Care, Neonatal—legislation &
jurisprudence—United States—Case Reports. WS 27 AA1 L296n 2006]
I. Meadow, William. II. Title.
RJ253.5.L37   2006
618.92′01—dc22   2005027715

A catalog record for this book is available from the British Library.

Contents

Acknowledgments   vii

1 Overview and Introduction   1

2 Some Facts about Infant Mortality and Neonatal Care   13

3 The Era of Innovation and Individualism, 1965–1982   18

4 The Era of Exposed Ignorance, 1982–1992   53

5 The End of Medical Progress, 1992 to the Present   85

6 Economics of the NICU   122

7 Four Discarded Moral Choices   136

8 The Possibility of Moral Progress   150

Notes   *159*
Index   *173*

Acknowledgments

The process by which a book comes into being is mysterious. This one began 15 years ago as a series of conversations and inquiries into the decision-making process in neonatal intensive care units. We began collecting data and presenting analyses at various scientific meetings, in particular the Society for Pediatric Research and the American Society of Bioethics and Humanities. Generous grant support from the Greenwall Foundation, the Robert Wood Johnson Foundation, and the MacLean Family helped continue the inquiries.

We have been fortunate to work at the University of Chicago, where Mark Siegler has created, in the MacLean Center for Clinical Medical Ethics, an extraordinary, feisty, and delightful group of colleagues, including Lainie Ross, Tracy Koogler, Jaideep Singh, Caleb Alexander, Farr Curlin, Stacy Lindau, Ann Dudley Goldblatt, Carol Stocking, Peter Smith, Alison Winter, and Dan Brudney. Over the years, conversations with Joel Frader, Jodi Halpern, Hilde Nelson, Carl Elliott, and Chris Feudtner have helped to refine our ideas.

Tom Murray at the Hastings Center and Wendy Harris of the Johns Hopkins University Press encouraged us to assemble these inquiries into a book. An anonymous reviewer helped us to shape the discussion and refine the arguments. William Silverman must be remembered as the guiding spirit behind all critical inquiries into neonatal bioethics. We miss him.

Neonatal Bioethics

CHAPTER ONE

Overview and Introduction

For the past half-century, the field of neonatology has grown and matured, like a baby in an incubator, in the strangely closed world of neonatal intensive care units (NICUs). Rarely have the processes and products of scientific medicine been as heralded and harangued, as lauded and condemned, as publicized and misunderstood as they have in the context of NICUs. In this book, we examine the creation and development of this particular field of modern medicine. By doing so, we try to understand something both about neonatology and, more generally, about the relationship between scientific progress, medical innovation, economics, bioethical reflection, and political regulation.

Neonatology is a good field to study in this way because it is one of the most successful medical innovations of the latter half of the twentieth century. It is an innovation without an innovator; that is, there was no "Eureka!" moment at which a key discovery brought the field into being. There was no particular individual who can be called the "founder of the field" or any particular time to which one can point as the first moment, the first success. Instead, a slow, synergistic accretion of different scientific and clinical insights, combined with an evolution in the way we build and shape the physical spaces of hospitals, changes in the way we finance medical care, and the elaboration and articulation of a moral stance toward the activities being developed, eventually led to something that might be called a new and separate field of medicine. Taken together, these interrelated endeavors have dramatically improved infant mortality rates throughout the world.

This process of innovation can be compared with medical innovations that developed in a different way. Examples of an alternative type of innovation abound. The discovery of insulin, penicillin, or polio vaccine comes to mind. In these cases, the individuals responsible can be identified, and the processes by which the innovations were discovered, tested, and incorporated into medical practice were fairly straightforward. Such innovations suggest a particular way of thinking about scientific progress. Because they were discrete and could be incorporated into existing structures of medical practice without altering those structures, such innovations reinforced, rather than challenged, prevailing notions of health, disease, health care, and the order of nature. They confirm the mechanistic view of such matters by which disease is a specific biochemical defect or can be remedied by a specific pharmacological agent. The agent's mechanism of action is delightfully straightforward and creates for the doctor a similarly straightforward role—applying the knowledge and deploying the technology.

In the late twentieth century, however, much medical innovation was of a different sort. With organ transplantation, cancer chemotherapy, or the treatment of coronary artery disease, complex infrastructures were created to elucidate the appropriate treatments, to test them, and to provide them. No individual, such as Alexander Fleming or Jonas Salk, can be identified as the discoverer of open-heart surgery or cancer chemotherapy. Instead, the discovery and deployment of these interventions required multiple trained personnel, a variety of technological devices, and an administrative structure to organize the complex interactions of people and machines. Neonatology is a prime example of this type of intervention. Understanding how it developed sheds light on common processes of medical innovation.

The decentralized and somewhat disorderly process by which innovation took place in neonatology and these other fields violated most rules and regulations for innovation in medicine that prevail today. Our examination of neonatal intensive care shows that the process of scientific progress and clinical innovation in such endeavors is different from the process on which many of the theoretical frameworks of medical ethics, health law, and health care financing are based. Innovative or experimental treatments can be identified as such under those frameworks and can then be carefully studied by comparing them to existing standard treatments to determine whether they are safe and effective. Once study of this kind has been completed, the treatments can be certified, licensed, or somehow recognized as no longer experimental. These treatments can then be incorporated into routine medical care. In an oversimplified way, this is the framework the Food and Drug Administration uses to evaluate a new drug.

The development of neonatal intensive care followed a different dynamic. Scientific and technological innovation was so rapid that important questions about the safety and efficacy of interventions could not be conceptualized until the scientific and technological innovations stimulated our imaginations to ask questions. The process of answering questions created new technologies, new understanding, and new questions, which could be answered only by further technological innovation. Along the way, and as an inherent part of the process (rather than as the starting point of the process), physicians and scientists learned how to ask the right questions. Articulating questions on the basis of new understanding engendered by exuberant innovation eventually led to consensus over what might qualify as an answer. Theoretical issues and practical issues, clinical and scientific issues, and moral, legal, and economic issues were thus inextricably intertwined, as were the treatments that were experimental, innovative, routine, and outdated.

In neonatology, as in many other fields of medicine with rapid innovation, treatments were introduced without careful research protocols and often without the meticulous informed consent of the research subjects. Thus, innovation sometimes violated conventional wisdom and public policy about the right way to conduct science, the legal way to innovate, and proper ethical norms. This is deeply troubling. However, whether the trouble is with innovators' behavior or with inadequate paradigms is unclear. Obedience to these prevailing research paradigms would almost certainly have protected some children from the harm that resulted from prematurely introducing poorly studied interventions. However, it would also have dramatically slowed the progress of neonatology and have led to the loss of thousands of babies whose lives were ultimately saved.

Critics and supporters of medical innovation thus face a difficult conundrum regarding neonatology: if today's rules and regulations governing clinical innovation are the proper rules, and if they might have prevented or slowed the development of one of the most successful medical innovations of modern medicine, then the cost of protection from risk is the slowing of progress. This conundrum has enormous implications for the future of biomedical innovation.

Each innovative field develops its own ethos as it progresses. That, too, is part of the story of neonatology. In the mid-1960s, as modern neonatology took shape, practitioners and observers recognized serious moral dilemmas in the activities of those who would use untested innovative treatments to try to save the lives of critically ill newborns. These practitioners and observers tried to articulate the dilemmas in a series of articles, books, and conference proceedings. Many of these initial forays into the uncharted moral territory of neonatology were conceptually confusing and factually naïve and ended in puzzlement more than in conviction.

Since then, rigorous philosophical inquiry, careful quantitative research, and a better understanding of the risks, benefits, and outcomes of neonatal care have led to a set of bioethical principles and practice parameters widely held and remarkably consistent around the world. These parameters define the terms of bioethical discourse about neonatology and allow discussion of the ethical issues and an agreed-upon range of both individual and cultural variation. Progress in neonatal bioethics is as remarkable as biomedical progress.

The medical successes of neonatology seem self-evident. Every year, in NICUs around the world, hundreds of thousands of babies are saved who, had they been born thirty or forty years ago, would have perished. In the United States, roughly 250,000 preterm infants are born each year. Before 1965, many of these babies would have died. Today, most survive. Furthermore, most survive without long-term health problems. Such success has made neonatology the largest subspecialty in pediatrics, and NICUs the cornerstone of every tertiary-care children's hospital in the United States.

But neonatology is not, of course, an unmitigated success. Although most babies treated in NICUs do well, many are left with lifelong medical problems. They survive with mild-to-severe chronic lung disease, visual impairment, seizures, or neurodevelopmental problems. Focus on these tragic outcomes of neonatal care has led some observers to conclude that neonatology is not one of the pinnacles of modern medical success but instead is one of the best examples of modern medicine's moral ambiguity or hubris.

One of the most moving and disturbing manifestations of these concerns is that some parents do not want NICU treatment for their critically ill babies. That is, they'd rather their baby die than be subjected to the hazards of neonatal intensive care. Carol Costellano, the mother of a premature baby, expressed these feelings, "If I'd had some way of knowing what (extremely premature) babies endure, I wouldn't have wanted my baby to go through that. I adore my daughter. I'd never wish her away. But if I were in premature labor, I wouldn't go to a hospital. I'd stay home and let nature take its course."[1] Ms. Costellano founded a support group for former preemies called Parents of Blind Children–New Jersey.

In 2000, a legal case in Texas pitted parents against the hospital in which their extremely premature, 23-week, 615-gram baby had been treated. The parents had asked that their baby not be resuscitated and instead be allowed to die. The doctors treated the baby anyway. The baby survived with severe impairments. A trial court awarded the parents $60 million, including $13.5 million in punitive damages. (This decision was later overturned on appeal.) Some commentators thought the trial court decision was the correct one. Jesuit priest and bioethicist John Paris wrote, "There comes a point with extremely premature infants . . . where the risk of mortality and morbidity becomes so significant and the degree of burden and the prospects of benefit so suffused in ambiguity and uncertainty that a decision as to whether to institute or continue medical treatment properly belongs to the parents."[2] Others thought the Texas Supreme Court was correct to reverse it. Lawyer and bioethicist George Annas wrote, "The Texas Supreme Court's decision limits physicians' discretion to the moments immediately after birth. The court does not require the neonatologist or obstetrician to treat or resuscitate a newborn, only to decide whether or not to treat or resuscitate newborns at birth. The Texas Supreme Court has made it clear that after the initial 'emergency' assessment, when many more treatment decisions must be made in the NICU, parental consent is legally required; if such consent is not forthcoming, a court order must be obtained before treatment proceeds. The narrow decision of the Texas Supreme Court was reasonable but nonetheless unfortunate for the Millers."[3] Such debates have surrounded neonatology since its inception.

These opposing interpretations of NICUs—modern miracle or medical nemesis—grip our collective moral imagination. Portrayals of NICUs in popular media amplify some of the myths that have grown up around them. The July 9, 1995, *New York Times Magazine* took readers inside the NICU of the Brigham and Women's Hospital of Harvard University. Author Darcy Frey describes the NICU thus: "It has the sleek, digitalized look of a space lab or, more nearly, a hydroponic tomato nursery." Such images suggest that the NICU combines the technologic aura of space exploration with that of agricultural biotechnology. The NICU is the place where the high-tech imagery of space missions meets the biotech imagery of genetically altered life forms. The babies themselves can be seen in such images as either passive, unheroic vegetables or dramatically adventurous astronauts.

Gayle Whittier recently reviewed the many metaphors that have been used to try to capture the realities of neonatal intensive care. She writes, "The dominant metaphor in and for the NICU, assigned by hospital personnel and lay persons alike, is that of extraterrestism and space exploration, the apotheosis of the technological future."[4] She also notes that military metaphors are commonly used.

Sometimes it is unclear whether the babies, the physicians, or the machines are the focus of the metaphors. If physicians are the space explorers, then what metaphoric role is left for the babies or the parents of those babies?

When the NICU is portrayed as a dangerous but seductive technology run amok, the professionals are seen as unreflective, unscientific, and irrational, motivated by their own rescue fantasies or by baser self-interests. Parents can reinforce this professional fantasy by seeing the NICU as a savior, a place where miracles will happen and babies are snatched from the jaws of death. Alternatively, they can see it as a place where they themselves and their babies are tortured, where they are systematically and perhaps even criminally deprived of the normal and appropriate rights that they, as parents, should have to make medical and moral decisions for their children.

Epidemiological studies of the long-term outcomes of NICU babies reflect the same sort of dichotomous responses, although the terms of the epidemiological debates are less picturesque. Nobody anymore doubts that NICUs improve the overall survival rates of critically ill babies. The debates focus, instead, on whether the survivors have such high rates of chronic health problems and developmental disabilities that they represent neonatology's Pyrrhic victory, creating more disease than would otherwise have been. The debate has been inconclusive. Some have concluded that the overall prevalence of cerebral palsy is increasing and that this is attributable to greater numbers of NICU survivors.[5] Others show that the prevalence of cerebral palsy has not changed.[6] Both sides in this debate agree on one thing: babies born at less than 28 weeks of gestation are at much higher risk of developing cerebral palsy or other neurological conditions than babies born at term. Because more such babies survive today than survived a generation ago, they account for a higher percentage of children with cerebral palsy than was once the case. In the past, cerebral palsy just happened. There was nothing we could do about it. Now it is associated, in many cases, with particular decisions about particular medical interventions that we can choose to use or to withhold. The overall prevalence of cerebral palsy may or may not have changed, but the moral responsibility and accountability felt by individuals for bad outcomes has clearly increased.

Arguments about the economics of NICUs are similarly heated. Neonatal intensive care has become the most expensive intervention in pediatrics. Before the advent of neonatology, it was inconceivable to spend hundreds of thousands of dollars to save a baby's life. Today, it has become both routine and routinely disturbing. From the beginning, questions have arisen about how NICUs should be funded, whether such treatment is cost effective, and whether NICUs siphon resources from other worthy programs and create need and dependency rather than health. Furthermore, because of the idiosyncrasies of health care financing rules, NICUs have become profit centers for many U.S. hospitals. This development raises a different set of concerns. Some worry that physicians and hospitals make decisions on the basis of the profitability of NICU treatment rather than for the best interests of the patients. Such arguments raise issues about distributive justice, economic conflicts of interest, and the effect of different methods of financing health care on clinical decision making.

For individuals who work in the NICU and for the parents of critically ill children, these complex abstract questions become concrete, immediate, and unavoidable. The care and treatment of each baby raises questions that must be answered with a specific decision or set of decisions. Should we initiate life-sustaining treatment? Who should decide? How much information is sufficient to be sure that parents understand the implications of the decisions they are being asked to make? Once initiated, when might treatment be stopped? How should those decisions be framed, explained, understood, acted on, or recovered from?

The focus on particular decisions for particular children, rather than on general questions about the fascinating philosophical, legal, or financial principles that ought to guide decisions, changes the moral focus of the decision. It is one thing to develop a philosophical rationale, a practice guideline, a legal framework, or a sophisticated cost-effectiveness analysis. It is quite another to watch a tiny baby struggle for breath, trying to decide whether particular treatments are likely to be more beneficial than harmful and trying to understand what it might mean for the baby and the family, or what it might tell us about ourselves, to make one choice over the other.

One well-recognized phenomenon shapes many decisions about the pros and cons of neonatal intervention: when parents are given the choice between trying a desperate treatment that has a small chance of short-term success or withholding treatment and letting their baby die, most parents choose treatment most of the time. The cases in which *either* a physician or a parent wants to withhold treatment are rare. The cases in which *both* physicians and parents agree that treatment should be withheld are rarer. The reasons for this phenomenon are multifaceted and have to do with epidemiology and emotions, with economics and politics, with religion and spirituality, and with the circumstances created by the collective cultural understandings about babies, parents, and medical care that have evolved over the past three decades.

The development of the science, technology, ethics, and economics of neonatology and NICUs has implications for other areas of medical development. NICUs are unique in many ways, but in other ways they are similar to or even emblematic of common aspects of medical innovation. Many moral questions central to modern medicine are raised to assess the development of neonatal intensive care. How should we innovate? How should we evaluate and regulate innovations? What sort of data should be incorporated into decisions? When do we know enough to deem an innovation standard and beneficial, rather than experimental? How should the benefits of expensive new therapies be fairly distributed? Who should pay? Who should profit? Who should decide? How do we find the proper balance among individual rights, collective obligations, and communal oversight?

These are complex, interlocking questions to which there are no simple answers. But answers should not be avoided. Just as the physician who attends to the birth of a premature baby must decide whether to initiate treatment, we as a society must choose how and when to regulate, support, or ignore medical innovations. We may designate some medical innovations as part of the vague entitlement that most Americans expect from certain forms of health care. Today, organ transplantation, renal dialysis, and cancer chemotherapy fit into this group. We may determine that certain innovations, such as psychotherapy, laser eye surgery, or in vitro fertilization, should be treated as free-market commodities. Other medical interventions, such as assisted suicide or reproductive cloning, might be prohibited.

This book describes the iterative, nonlinear, and, sometimes, heated process by which the answers to moral, legal, economic, and political questions evolved in neonatology, a process that involved multiple stakeholders and constituencies. Modes of discourse as varied as public health reports, philosophical and theological analyses, and tort litigation were required and evoked conceptual feedback loops among various constituencies. Overlap sometimes led to incoherence. At certain junctures, the passion and the blindness of the innovators met the hopes and fears of parents and the political interests of judges or legislators in a combustible combination.

To bring some descriptive clarity to this long and complex process, we divide the development of neonatal intensive care into three different eras. The first era began with the introduction of mechanical ventilation for premature babies in the late 1960s and lasted until the early 1980s. During this era, many physicians and health care administrators understood that they were engaged in a vast, uncontrolled medical, moral, social, and economic experiment. They struggled to understand the meaning of the experiment and its implications for the practice of medicine. Many physicians were frightened of the new technology and of their role as purveyors of it. They raised important questions about whether we were doing more harm than good by trying to save sicker and sicker babies.

This was also the era of some of neonatology's most dramatic successes, when medical professionals and society first recognized neonatal intensive care as a bona fide subspecialty of medical work. This led to the creation of a subspecialty board in neonatology in 1975. Legislation establishing regionalized perinatal networks and designated referral centers for the care of the sickest babies were also established. These organizational infrastructures allowed NICUs to develop into their present form. They also allowed investigators to begin asking the questions that would shape the development of the field.

The second era began with a legal controversy over a case in which a baby with

Down syndrome ("Baby Doe") was allowed to die rather than undergo lifesaving surgery. The case stimulated federal regulations that reinterpreted the moral problems of neonatal intensive care. Before Baby Doe, many people feared the overuse of therapies that had not been carefully evaluated. The Baby Doe regulators, by contrast, suggested that the central problem might be the underuse of proven therapies based on inappropriate assessments of the baby's quality of life. The goal of the regulations was to develop a consistent national standard for such decisions to replace the decentralized and individualized model that prevailed in the first era.

The proposed federal regulations were eventually invalidated. Nevertheless, they had, and still have, enormous symbolic power. They represented a consensus statement about the type of concerns and considerations that ought to guide decision making for newborns. The process of developing this consensus statement forced physicians to confer with lawyers, parents, and advocates for people with disabilities and to question prevailing professional habits. This process uncovered previously unrecognized or misunderstood disagreements about the role of physicians, the preferences of parents, the limits of parental discretion, and the use of quality-of-life assessments. It forced physicians to consider ways in which any standardizing regulations might be implemented. For example, the Baby Doe criteria permitted the withdrawal of "futile" or "inhumane" treatment, but they did not define "futility" or "inhumanity." Research and discussion would clarify the meaning of these words and allow people to use them in day-to-day experience.

During this era, certain assumptions about parents, nurses, and doctors were reexamined. In the 1970s, many people worried that doctors, driven by a technological imperative, would inappropriately *impose* treatment on babies that would lead to survivors with an unacceptable quality of life. One of the surprises of the Baby Doe controversy, for pediatricians and neonatologists, was that they were being accused of a different sort of paternalism. They were criticized for inappropriately *withholding* treatments that parents might have wanted and of unjustly judging quality of life as unacceptable or intolerable. Nobody was clear precisely how to quantify or to respond to these sorts of transgressions. Before the late 1980s, there were no data to suggest which set of attitudes or which sort of decision-making dynamic was more common.

These concerns ushered in the third era of neonatal ethics. To answer questions raised by the attempts to develop national standards, researchers undertook different sorts of studies. The creation of multicenter databases to examine neonatal practices and outcomes created a knowledge base about common practices and practice variations. Researchers asked parents what they really wanted. They studied physicians' prognostic abilities. They quantified variations in practice. These databases allowed physicians and researchers to quantify medical progress by examining changes in survival rates over time. Such studies showed that, by the mid-1990s, medical progress in neonatology began to slow or even stop.

The end of rapid, steady medical progress in neonatology has important moral implications. Throughout the 1970s and 1980s, neonatology led to continual improvements in outcomes for babies. As long as such progress continued, prognostication was difficult because the long-term outcome studies that would help with prognostication were obsolete by the time they were complete. By the mid-1990s, however, as survival rates began to level off, prognostic accuracy improved. Physicians no longer had to modify data from the recent past to account for the as-yet-unmeasured effects of recent innovations. Perhaps unsurprisingly, the focus of legal regulation shifted from the legislative arena to the malpractice courtroom as attorneys, judges, and juries grappled with what was or should be the standard of medical care in an arena that was becoming increasingly standardized.

Together, these developments in the third era of modern neonatology have allowed the development of a fairly consistent set of decision-making criteria and policies. These criteria allow physicians to characterize clinical situations as ones in which outcomes are predictably good enough that treatment is considered mandatory or as ones in which outcomes are uncertain enough or bleak enough that treatment is considered optional. In making these judgments, physicians consider both the chances for survival and the anticipated quality of life. These criteria are not immutable. Many people are deeply troubled by some features of the current consensus. Nevertheless, these criteria have led to a relative quiescence in the number of cases in which moral uncertainty becomes so paralyzing that participants are stumped about how to proceed. Such cases used to be far more common in neonatal intensive care.

Our vision of neonatology today, then, is different from many popular portrayals of the field. The NICU is often portrayed as a frontier filled with cataclysmic struggles fought by heroic crusaders against implacable biological constraints, with tiny human infants as the battleground. Mostly, it is not. Instead, today's NICU is a surprisingly mundane place that runs like a happy factory, churning out healthy baby after healthy baby, with mostly routine efforts by highly trained professionals. Undeniably, dramatic and morally charged events occur, including agonizing decisions about whether to continue treatment; however, they do not occur very often, and when they do, they are dealt with in a systematized and relatively standardized way.

For the remainder of this book, we will detail the substance of controversies in each of these different eras. Our method is both historical and philosophical. Our primary interest is the changes in societal moral attitudes about medical treatment for babies and the role of physicians and parents in deciding which babies should and should not be treated.

To orient readers to our discussion of these issues, we will first provide an overview of facts and trends regarding infant mortality in the United States in the twentieth century. We will then discuss these three different eras in some detail, describing the medical advances of the era, the epidemiological discoveries, the shifts in health policy and medical economics, and the legal changes. The dominant ethical approaches and legal responses of each era are reconstructed.

Our approach does not involve primary data collection. We will use existing primary sources—articles in scholarly journals and in newspapers and magazines—to illustrate what was reported about beliefs and practices during these times. Thus, we are not doing the sort of social science research that scholars such as Renee Anspach,[7] Myra Bluebond-Langner, or Jeanne Guillieman and Lynda Holmstrom have done. These scholars' books are part of the existing data that we examine to construct our overview.

One potential drawback of our approach is that these secondary sources may not accurately reflect actual practices. In some instances, dramatic cases may garner a lot of attention and highlight certain features of the moral dilemmas in neonatology that are emotionally charged but not common. In some cases, detailed study of practices at one or two hospitals may show the approaches of particular physicians or a particular institution but in a way that makes it difficult to determine whether those physicians or institutions are representative or idiosyncratic. In other instances, physicians may portray their own behavior and practices in a manner that is colored by memory, idealism, or fear of litigation. However, this is not meant to be a new study of the actual practices of any particular physician or any one NICU. Instead, it is meant to be an overview of the development of the field over the past thirty years. Although we rely on secondary data sources, we also draw on our own experiences as practitioners, as members of a busy hospital ethics consultation service, and as people who have visited neonatal units around the world and talked to doctors, nurses, and parents about their experiences. In the end, this approach leads to reflections and conclusions that are both personal and somewhat idiosyncratic. Their ultimate value will rest not on our methodological rigor but on the reader's intuition about the validity of our observations.

At the end of the book, we will discuss the implications of the development of ethics in the NICU for other situations in which biomedical advances create new moral dilemmas. We will conclude that neonatal bioethics has been as much of a success story as neonatal medicine. Taken together, they create a paradigm of medical and bioethical progress that might inform other contentious areas. The keys to that progress have been responsible professional leadership; carefully crafted legislation that provides appropriate infrastructure, oversight, and accountability; recognition of both knowledge and ignorance; and open dialogue between scientists, clinicians, ethicists, legislators, and regulators. We hope that our analysis of this model will be useful to reflect on as we face dilemmas in other areas of biomedical innovation.

CHAPTER TWO

Some Facts about Infant Mortality and Neonatal Care

Neonatal mortality is defined as death before 28 days of age. Postneonatal mortality is defined as death between 28 days and 1 year. Infant mortality is the sum of these two and is defined as death before 1 year of age.

When these mortality rates are reported, they are usually offered for different groups of babies, classified by birthweight. Babies who weigh less than 2500 grams (5.5 pounds) at birth are classified as low birthweight. Babies who weigh less than 1500 grams (3.3 pounds) at birth are considered very low birthweight. In some reports, another category, extremely low birth weight, describes outcomes for babies who weigh less than 1000 grams (2.2 pounds) at birth.

Infant mortality rates are generally reported not as percentages but as deaths per 1000 live births.

Gestational maturity is highly correlated with birthweight, but some premature babies are larger than average and so fall within the range of normal for birthweight, while some full-term babies are smaller than average and hence of low birthweight. The numbers of babies in these two groups are relatively small, so, generally speaking, low birthweight means premature.

In the United States, infant mortality has dropped from 55/1000 in 1900 to 9/1000 in 2000. Trends over the century reveal much about the reasons for the improvement. In the early part of the century, the improvement was in both neonatal and postneonatal mortality. Most epidemiologists attribute these improvements to public health measures, such as better nutrition and sanitation. In the mid-twentieth century, postneonatal mortality rates improved faster than neonatal mortality rates.

This is usually attributed to medical interventions such as antibiotics and immunizations that had greater efficacy in older babies than in neonates.

In 1960, the neonatal mortality rate in the United States was 19/1000. It steadily dropped over the next decades, to 16 in 1970, 13 in 1980, 9 in 1990, and 4 in 2000. Much of the recent drop is attributable to improvements in survival for low birthweight babies. These improvements in birthweight-specific neonatal mortality are generally attributed to improvements in neonatal intensive care and, in particular, in the care of tiny premature babies.[1]

Many of the patients in NICUs are premature babies, but there are two other groups of babies who are admitted to NICUs, full-term babies with acute illness and babies with congenital anomalies. These other groups of NICU patients are both medically and ethically distinct.

THREE GROUPS OF BABIES WHO ARE ADMITTED TO NICUS

Overall, three relatively distinct groups of babies are admitted to neonatal intensive care units. The first group is *full-term or near-term babies with acute illnesses* such as pneumonia or sepsis or babies with surgically correctable anatomic abnormalities. The second group comprises *babies with congenital anomalies* that are not correctable at present. These include chromosomal anomalies such as Down syndrome. Many of these babies have problems that can be ameliorated but not fully corrected with surgical or medical treatment. The third group comprises those *babies born prematurely* who are otherwise physically normal; that is, they have no acute illness or congenital anomaly except prematurity. These groups of babies raise different clinical and ethical issues. It is important to recognize these three groups and to understand their differences because, to the extent that we think about all babies admitted to the NICU as relatively similar, we miss important differences that form the basis of our ethical responses.

Full-term babies with acute illnesses are usually the least morally controversial. Most acute illnesses can be treated if they are accurately diagnosed. The problems that arise in decision making for such babies are similar to the problems related to other high-risk patients of any age—diagnoses must be made quickly and treatment initiated expeditiously. Time or need for discussion is limited. The medical indications for treatment define the moral obligations for treatment. These babies generally either get better quickly or die quickly. Ethical problems arise only when treatment is partially successful and the babies survive but with severe long-term complications of their acute illness. For example, full-term babies might develop meningitis, be diagnosed and treated, but then be left with a severe neurological impairment or dependence on medical technology for survival. At that point, the ethical issues are similar to those of babies born with congenital anomalies, namely, questions about quality of life and the relative benefits and burdens of continued treatment.

Babies with congenital anomalies are the second group of babies who often require neonatal intensive care. These babies were the primary focus of legal and moral controversy in the 1970s regarding treatment decisions for newborns. In particular, discussion focused on syndromes such as trisomy 21 (Down syndrome), spina bifida, and multiple congenital malformations. In general, the ethical issues that arise in the care of these babies focus on whether to provide life-sustaining intensive care or corrective surgical treatment that will treat or ameliorate one problem but not the underlying congenital syndrome. Thus, for babies with Down syndrome, the issue may be whether to correct an intestinal or cardiac malformation. In babies with spina bifida, it may be whether to treat the hydrocephalus by placing a shunt in the brain or whether to close the open lesion of the spinal canal, the defining feature of the syndrome. The essence of these dilemmas is that (1) the underlying syndromes cannot not be cured; (2) treatment of the life-threatening manifestations is generally feasible and successful; (3) babies who are successfully treated will be left with significant impairments of one sort or another; and (4) if these life-threatening manifestations are not treated, then "nature will take its course" and the babies will die. In such a situation, many people think that sometimes, depending on the precise facts, letting nature take its course and allowing the baby to die is preferable to medical or surgical intervention.

Controversies about the treatment of babies with congenital anomalies thus focus discussion on the baby's anticipated quality of life as opposed to prognosis for survival. They force us to ask whether there are situations in which it is medically possible to save a baby's life but ethically unwise to do so because that life will be so problematic in some way that the baby would be better off dead. These controversies became the focus of the Baby Doe controversy in the 1980s. They will be discussed in more detail in Chapter 4.

Babies with extreme prematurity comprise the third group of babies admitted to the NICU. The moral considerations for these babies include all of the considerations in the other two but add an important new one—long-term prognostic uncertainty.

Prematurity is both an acute crisis and a chronic condition. The acute crisis requires an emergency response driven by medical indications, just as in the cases of full-term babies with acute medical problems. At the time when treatment is initiated, however, the baby's prognosis is usually uncertain in a different way than for the other two situations. With acute pneumonia, for example, treatment will likely either succeed, in which case there will be complete resolution of the problem, or it will fail, in which case the baby will die. There is almost no middle ground. With congenital anomalies and syndromes, treatment cannot cure the underlying disease but will almost surely be successful in treating some of the associated conditions. Thus, the long-term prognosis for survivors in such cases is clearly predictable. Again, there is almost no middle ground of prognostic uncertainty.

With extremely premature babies, by contrast, the prognosis is radically uncertain. For any given baby, the potential outcomes range from early death to late death to survival with severe, moderate, or mild disabilities, to survival with no long-term medical or neurodevelopmental problems. Furthermore, the disabilities associated with the "disease" can be cognitive, pulmonary, intestinal, or cardiac or involve virtually any other organ system. At the time when treatment must be initiated, nearly all of these babies are in a situation of radical prognostic uncertainty. Doctors cannot say what the outcome for any particular baby will be. Instead, the range of possibilities covers the spectrum of outcomes, from the very best to the very worst. Doctors in these situations usually give parents probabilistic estimates. For example, they might say that a baby has a 50 percent chance of survival and that, among survivors, 30 percent are severely disabled. Such numbers, though accurate, are not helpful in the way that the prognostic estimates in cases of acute illness or congenital syndromes are helpful. They do not indicate with any precision the expected outcome for the individual baby. Instead, they merely quantify the radical uncertainties and describe a range of possibilities. This radical uncertainty raises another set of ethical considerations.

In these cases, the key question focuses on the degree of certainty that must be achieved before various moral thresholds are crossed. One moral threshold defines situations in which treatment is morally and legally obligatory. If the prognosis is good enough, then parents are not permitted to refuse intervention. Instead, the decision to treat is driven by an assessment of what is in the best interest of the baby. In most NICUs, babies born after 25 weeks of gestation are in this category. A second threshold is when the outcomes are probabilistically bad, so that treatment might be considered morally and legally optional. In those cases, parents are given the facts as straightforwardly and accurately as possible and are allowed to make a decision one way or the other—to continue or to discontinue life-sustaining treatment. Babies born between 23 and 25 weeks of gestation are in this category. A third threshold is one in which survival is unprecedented or treatment is futile. Babies who are born before 23 weeks generally fall into this category. However, these categories are only the starting points for decision making. We offer them here only as an illustration of the theoretical framework by which morally obligatory, morally permissible, and morally prohibited thresholds might be conceptualized. We explore them in more detail in Chapter 5.

These trends in infant mortality, facts about the clinical epidemiology of neonatal care, and overview of the typology of moral considerations set the framework for understanding the historical development of neonatal intensive care and clinical decision making for critically ill newborns that is the focus of this book. With these overall patterns, trends, and categories in mind, we will now examine in more detail the changes in attitudes, practices, regulations, and financing that occurred over the past three decades that led to current understandings of the implications of medical progress for the treatment of critically ill newborns.

CHAPTER THREE

The Era of Innovation and Individualism, 1965–1982

The story of clinical innovation in medicine is often frightening. It involves a certain degree of hubris. Innovators must think that they can use science, cleverness, and narcissistic grandiosity to improve on tradition. Such adventures often end badly. They are usually stories of fits and starts; of irrational exuberance and of avoidable tragedy; of skill, luck, science, and serendipity. Sometimes, they involve glaring moral lapses or even criminal activity. Many innovators are not recognized or rewarded for their work. Some are lionized.

Such stories are often transformed, in retrospect, into more orderly narratives that are almost fictional in the way they reconstruct the process of innovation. The story of the "discovery" of penicillin is a good example of such a mythologizing transformation of the facts. In the parable that schoolchildren learn, Alexander Fleming's fortuitous recognition of the therapeutic potential of the bacteria-killing mold on one of his petri dishes led directly to the clinical develop of an antimicrobial wonder drug. There is in this, as in all myths, a grain of truth. The development of antimicrobial agents that could be used to treat life-threatening infections clearly changed the course of medical history and world history, though that process did not really begin with Fleming and penicillin. Furthermore, the process by which penicillin got from Fleming's petri dish to clinical use was far more complicated than this story suggests.

His accidental discovery, in 1928, was reported in 1929. However, he was unable to take the next step. He never figured out how to purify significant quantities of the chemical that he named "penicillin," so he was unable to test it clinically. He gave up work on the substance in 1931 and, if that had been the end of the story, penicillin might be remembered as an agent that could interfere with the proper culture of bacteria in the laboratory.

Ten years later, Howard Florey, Ernst Chain, and Norman Heatley discovered ways to overcome the technical difficulties that stumped Fleming. They began to produce penicillin in large enough quantities to use clinically. Their purification process was so cumbersome and expensive that, although they were able to use it clinically, they did not have enough to treat more than a few patients. However, they did achieve dramatic and tantalizing success in the treatment of pneumonia. The Nobel Prize committee recognized that their contribution was at least as significant as Fleming's and awarded the 1945 Nobel Prize in Physiology or Medicine to Fleming, Florey, and Chain. In his acceptance speech, Florey described the "immense amount of work" that had been done on antibiotics over the preceding sixty years.[1]

A few years later, Albert Elder and Robert Coghill, working in Peoria, Illinois, used a variant strain of Fleming's penicillin that had been discovered on a cantaloupe in a Peoria fruit market as the basis for a new process that allowed efficient production of large quantities of penicillin.[2] This process, spurred by the war effort and jointly funded by the government and a consortium of drug companies, made commercial use of the drug practical. By D-day, they had produced 300 billion units of the wonder drug. Thus, it took nearly two decades and dozens of scientists on two continents to transform Fleming's initial observations into a drug with true clinical applicability.

As with many medical innovations, penicillin solved some problems, created others, and opened whole new avenues for investigation. Other antibiotics were discovered, bacteria developed resistance to many of them, the treatment of infectious diseases changed radically as the balance of efficacy shifted back and forth between the newer antibiotics and the newer forms of bacterial resistance. In addition to these biochemical and pharmacological problems, there were ethical and economic problems. The availability of drugs that could treat previously life-threatening infections allowed doctors to "play God" in whole new ways. William Osler had viewed pneumonia as "the old man's friend" because it was sometimes the mechanism by which chronically ill or debilitated patients died.[3] With the advent of antibiotic therapy, such patients frequently survived. Sometimes, survival seemed worse than death. Decisions now had to be made about whether interventions to prevent death were the right thing to do. Penicillin was one of the first interventions that made death something that had to be chosen, rather than something that simply occurred.

The complex and collective process by which penicillin went from laboratory bench to clinical bedside and then by which the risks, benefits, indications, contraindications, promise, and peril of the innovation came to be understood is the norm in medical innovation. For advances that involve something more than a single drug, the process becomes even more complicated. Most such efforts fail. The ones that succeed are remembered and create a sanitized version of the history of medical progress.

Innovation in neonatology is filled with examples of efforts that did not quite work out as promised. For example, if one looks at the process by which supplemental oxygen therapy for neonatal respiratory distress syndrome was tried, widely adopted, criticized, studied, modified, and studied again, one sees the whole dynamic of neonatal innovation in microcosm. Silverman recently summarized key points in this history, highlighting the following milestones:

1942	Investigators in Michigan show that irregular respirations in premature babies can be converted to regular respirations if the babies are given supplemental oxygen.
Mid-1940s	Newly designed incubators using molded plastics make it possible to maintain high concentrations of oxygen for prolonged periods of time.
1951	Mary Crosse, in Birmingham, investigates the cause of a new type of infantile blindness—retinopathy of prematurity—and suspects that excess oxygen exposure might be the cause.
1952	Patz and Hoeck conduct an alternate assignment, parallel treatment trial of high- versus low-oxygen regimens. Their results implicate high-dose oxygen as a cause of retinopathy.
1953	A conference is held in Bethesda about whether and how to study the issue. One group thinks a clinical trial of supplemental oxygen is essential. Another group thinks a clinical trial would be unethical because the data linking high-dose oxygen with retinopathy are already so compelling. The trialists prevail. A multicenter trial is initiated.
1954	Results of multicenter trial show that there was no appreciable increase in mortality for babies who received a lower dose of oxygen. Oxygen curtailment led to a two-thirds reduction in eye disease.
1960	A reanalysis of the data from the trial suggests methodological flaws. In particular, it appears that the mortality rate in the low-oxygen group was much higher than previously reported. One analysis suggested that there were sixteen

	excess deaths for every case of retinopathy prevented. The optimum dose of oxygen to give babies remains unclear.
1960s–1970s	With the development of better laboratory techniques, attention shifts from the level of oxygen provided to the baby to the partial pressure of oxygen in the baby's blood. No prospective studies are carried out, though. Instead, results of retrospective studies are used to develop consensus recommendations for treatment.
1980s–1990s	New techniques for mechanical ventilation are tried, including high-frequency oscillatory ventilation[4] and liquid ventilation. Some appear beneficial. Others appear likely only to delay the process of dying without improving rates of survival.
Twenty-first century	Randomized trial of high- versus low-oxygen saturation shows no difference in mortality or developmental outcomes.

From this history, Silverman concludes, "There has never been a shred of convincing evidence to guide limits for the rational use of supplemental oxygen in the care of extremely premature infants. For decades, the optimum range of oxygenation (to balance four competing risks: mortality, retinopathy of prematurity with blindness, chronic lung disease, and brain damage) was, and remains to this day, unknown."[5] Silverman overstates the case. It is not that there has never been a shred of evidence but that, instead, there have been many shreds of sometimes contradictory evidence, many efforts to balance the demands of clinical care with those of careful research, and many moral tensions created by the perceived imbalances that arose between the two. Any particular new study, no matter how well designed, would not clear up this confusion. If anything, it might add to it by providing one more thread of evidence to be woven into an already complex tapestry.

This brief summary of the complex history of the use of oxygen in neonates suggests how new clinical interventions evolve. They begin with an insight or idea. This leads some pioneers to change their clinical practices. Science, clinical experience, the perceptions of ethical obligations, the economic climate, and luck can all lead some practitioners to shift their ideas, while others hold fast to less innovative ways of practicing. Dogma sometimes becomes rigid before studies are conclusive. Responsible investigators are sometimes lauded and sometimes pilloried. Moral obligations can be asserted both for carrying out controlled further studies before adopting an innovation into standard practice and for not carrying out such trials. Somehow, out of the mix, change happens. Some practices are adopted, others are abandoned, and still others are put on the back burner, awaiting further study or new technological innovations. The process has implications for the way we think about both science and ethics and for the way we think about the intersection between the two in the practice of medicine.

A traditional and comforting way to conceptualize the intersection between scientific inquiry and ethical oversight of medical science is to draw a bright line between "clinical practice" and "clinical research." By this conceptual approach, we understand "clinical practice" to be a set of activities based on what is *known*. This knowledge leads to widely accepted standards of care. Doctors are bound by their professional moral obligations and by the law to uphold those standards. Patients are asked to give their informed consent for treatment, a process guided by legal rules about disclosure of risks. There is no prospective oversight of the informed consent process, only the possibility of retrospective review and punishment if the process is later judged to have been negligent. Under this rubric, only the clinician decides which options should or should not be offered to the patient and which risks to disclose.

By this same conceptual approach, we understand "clinical research" to be a set of activities that focuses on new, innovative, or experimental clinical interventions. Physician-investigators, in theory, understand what is known and distinguish it from what is unknown. Patients who are participants in clinical trials are seen as requiring special layers of protection. Special research review committees scrutinize the research protocols, fine-tune the informed consent documents, and carefully monitor the trials for adverse events. When a clinical research protocol is complete, the innovative therapy's effectiveness will be judged based on careful scientific analysis and will then either be incorporated into clinical practice or discarded.

Even a cursory reading of the history of neonatology (or, for that matter, of most other innovative fields of medicine) will show that this idealized process bears little resemblance to reality. The disjunction between the theory of innovation and reality is important because theory often informs policy in a way that tries to nudge reality closer to the theoretical ideal. Sometimes, this is appropriate. Sometimes, theory is so clearly preferable and reality so clearly deficient that the need for regulatory interventions to reform practices is compelling. At other times, however, it is less clear whether theory is so clearly superior to practice. The very nature of reflective practice, which is to say good practice, is that practitioners incorporate unarticulated (and sometimes even unconceptualized) theoretical concerns into their activities in ways that make the divide between theory and practice indistinct.

To better understand the actual process of innovation within neonatal intensive care, we will look in some detail at the development of two of the key innovations that made modern neonatal intensive care possible: mechanical ventilation and total parenteral nutrition (TPN). Our examination of the development of these innovations will focus on the tensions between scientific rigor, clinical practice, and public presentation. We are less interested in the quality of the science itself than in the way that barriers are crossed in the initial use of therapies, the initial presentation of results, and the eventual incorporation of these innovations into clinical practice.

THE DEVELOPMENT OF MECHANICAL VENTILATION

As background, these innovations were both pioneered in the 1960s. This was an era of unprecedented innovation in neonatology. By contrast, the preceding three decades had been relatively unadventurous. Between 1922, when Chicago pediatrician Julius Hess opened a twenty-eight-bed "incubator station" in Chicago, and 1963, when President Kennedy's 2-day-old son died of hyaline membrane disease in a hyperbaric oxygen chamber in Boston, clinical innovations in the field improved the survival of full-term babies but did little for babies born prematurely.

In 1963, as in 1922, premature babies died primarily from two causes. Either they had diseases of the lungs associated with prematurity, or they were unable to get enough nutrition through their immature intestinal tracts. Until these basic problems could be addressed, all other interventions commonly used before 1965—supplemental oxygen, temperature control, treatment of infections, and exchange transfusion for the treatment of hyperbilirubinemia—primarily benefited full-term (or nearly full-term) babies.

By the late 1950s, physicians and scientists began to understand that the primary cause of respiratory distress in premature babies was the lack of pulmonary surfactant, a substance that allows the lungs to inflate more easily with each breath. This discovery led to a shift in therapeutic focus. Doctors realized that the approach at that time of simply providing supplemental oxygen failed because surfactant deficiency made it impossible for the lungs to use the oxygen. Instead, babies needed something to keep their pulmonary alveoli from collapsing with each breath. Two solutions were proposed. One was to develop a pharmaceutical version of surfactant. That approach came to fruition later. The other was to not just provide oxygen but to provide it under enough distending pressure to expand the surfactant-deficient lungs of premature babies. The hope was that such pressure-supported breathing would be more effective than mere oxygen enrichment.

The search for the proper way to provide that pressure support was the search that led to the development of modern neonatal intensive care. In fact, the modern era of neonatology began with the introduction of intermittent positive pressure ventilation for newborn babies who had respiratory distress syndrome. This innovation was a process rather than an event, a sustained collective effort rather than an individual revelation. Different doctors at different centers in different countries tried different techniques to assist newborns with life-threatening respiratory failure.

The earliest reports of the use of positive-pressure ventilation were full of wonder, awe, fear, and excitement. Delivoria-Papadopoulos, Levison, and Swyer, physicians at the Research Institute of the Hospital for Sick Children in Toronto, published one of the first reports of successful treatment of the disease that they called "severe respiratory distress syndrome" in newborns using a treatment they called "intermittent positive pressure respiration," or IPPR. Although this was one of the first reports of such treatment in a peer-reviewed medical journal, they (like the developers of penicillin) noted in their introduction that they were building on previous scientific reports, including their own previous work, describing the successful use of similar therapies.

In a previous publication, they had "demonstrated the possibility of reversing at least temporarily the biochemical changes of terminal asphyxia in patients dying with RDS."[6] That carefully worded phrase suggests the first problem that these innovators faced. They were not quite sure how to define success. They were, remember, working at the end of a decade in which the "success" or "failure" or supplemental oxygen therapy had been a subject of vigorous public and professional debate. It was a time of optimism but also of cautious, guarded optimism.

"Success" in the use of IPPR might not necessarily mean the survival of the patient. Instead, it may mean that the technique itself is shown to be feasible and physiologically effective even if it is not clinically beneficial to the patient. (This is, by the way, similar to the penicillin story, in which the first clinical trial in a human patient was successful only in slowing the course of the disease. Eventually, they ran out of penicillin and the patient died.) This distinction between what might be called physiological success and what might be called clinical success remains a crucial and central concept of both the epidemiology and ethics of neonatal intensive care. Now, as then, some treatments can be shown to have positive physiological effects long before they are shown to have desirable clinical outcomes.

Delivoria-Papadopoulos and colleagues moved from physiologic feasibility to possible clinical usefulness by making a change in the clinical indications for using mechanical ventilation. In their article, they write, "Previous experience of assisting ventilation, begun only after repeated resuscitative attempts by bagging had failed, yielded only 1 survivor out of 19. In our present series assisted ventilation was started *as soon as it was obvious* [emphasis added] that mask bagging would be ineffective in restoring sustained respiration. Thus infants did not deteriorate over many hours as in our previous series." In a sense, this approach represents the flip side of the problem of defining success: defining failure. The only justification for attempting an innovative therapy with unknown risks was if the standard therapy had failed (or could be reliably predicted to fail). It is not always clear, or obvious, when that point is reached. A primary task of an innovator is to recognize such failures in new ways.

Because such seemingly minor innovations would become a hallmark of neonatal innovation that this one is worth examining in some detail. The key question that one might ask is how it became "obvious" to these investigators that mask bagging would not work for a particular baby. In other words, how did they know, or come to believe, that the standard treatment of the day would be ineffective? They do not say, precisely, in the published report.

We know that Dr. Delivoria-Papadopoulos was a pioneer in the development of techniques of tracheal intubation. She was eager to try this new technique on newborns. We also know that many of the other doctors in her hospital, and most doctors in other hospitals, were reluctant to allow this sort of unproven therapy for babies. Remember that her initial work in Toronto was being carried out at a time when leading centers in the United States, such as Boston Children's Hospital, were still relying on hyperbaric oxygen, even for a child of the U.S. president. In Toronto, Delivoria-Papadopoulos was initially not allowed to try IPPR until all other efforts at resuscitation had failed. In essence, her initial (and unpublished) work in this clinical area was carried out on babies who had already died. At that point, when all else had failed, she would be allowed to intubate babies and give IPPR. She discovered that some of the babies could actually be "brought back to life" for a short period of time. These bizarre, unreported early experiences were the foundation on which reported clinical trials were eventually based.[7]

The change that the Toronto investigators made in their clinical approach to these critically ill babies—a change in the time of initiation of IPPR—can be thought about in a number of ways. One way would be to use the language of clinical research trials and to think of it as a change in the "eligibility criteria" for the trial. In any clinical trial, the researchers must decide what clinical condition or set of physiologic or pathologic indicators makes one eligible to be a subject in the trial. In this case, their previous eligibility criterion for IPPR was that one had to have undergone bag and mask ventilation for at least two hours without improvement. Such a strict criterion would protect patients from the risk of the innovative therapy (IPPR) until the innovators were fairly certain that they would not benefit from the standard therapy (bag and mask ventilation). However, it also created an implicit impediment to the success of the innovative therapy because only babies who were so moribund as to be virtually unsalvageable would be eligible for the clinical trial.

If, however, they were to relax the eligibility criteria, they could allow patients into the clinical trial of mechanical ventilation who might, in fact, have survived without it. Those would be the patients for whom bag and mask ventilation might have worked if it had only been given a chance but who now, instead, would be offered the potential benefits and also be exposed to the unknown risks of the innovative therapy. The judgment to change the eligibility criteria was a judgment that the innovative therapy, IPPR, was safe enough so that it was ethically acceptable to expose infants to its risks even if they might not have needed it for survival.

Judgments about eligibility criteria are, essentially, decisions about who should be the experimental guinea pigs—who should go first. Most people do not want to be guinea pigs. Most parents do not want their children to be experimented on. Nevertheless, progress is impossible without innovation or experimentation. Those who go first face the risks of innovation that generate benefits for others. Selection criteria are necessary, are inevitable, and always have a tragic element. Blameless individuals are exposed to potential suffering so that others, someday, might not suffer.

One cultural-psychological response to the conflict between the desire for progress and the abhorrence of experimentation in medicine is to imagine that what is going on is not, in fact, experimenting at all. Instead, innovators tell themselves they are using their best critical and clinical judgment to provide the best treatment for each baby, even if the best treatment is a treatment that has just been invented and about which they know little. By this rationale, they are able to conceptually and morally place their work in the domain of innovative therapy rather than research or experimentation and to proceed under the less rigorous ethical guidelines that govern clinical treatment rather than the more rigorous ones that govern clinical research.

But is this rationale valid? What happens if we reconceptualize the innovations of the Toronto group as an attempt to define eligibility criteria for a clinical trial? The task of defining eligibility criteria for any clinical trial has embedded within it complicated moral and epidemiologic judgments about the relative risks and benefits of "standard" and "experimental" treatments. Such decisions are inevitably both moral and scientific. The uncertainty associated with them can be *reduced* by careful science and by objective reasoning but it cannot be *eliminated*. In the end, a moral judgment must be made about whether the inevitably unknown risks to a particular patient, a particular baby, a particular research subject, are worth the inevitably unquantifiable potential benefits.

Because such moral judgments are inevitably disturbing, researchers try to displace or disguise them. They can be reframed as technical discussions about the ap-

propriate design of the clinical experiment. When the experiment is part of a formal clinical trial, with a defined study question, rigorous methodology, and a plan
for the statistical analysis of the results, the value judgments inherent in the decisions about eligibility can be identified, scrutinized, and modified. When, instead,
as is often the case in areas of clinical innovation, the eligibility criteria are constantly shifting and the evaluation is not so much a process of testing a hypothesis
as it is a process of retrospectively evaluating a set of experiences, the distinctions
get blurred. What we are calling "eligibility criteria" may come to be defined, or refined, after the fact rather than before.

Looked at in this way, the complex process of clinical innovation that took place
in the earliest clinical trials of assisted ventilation in neonatology can be seen as a
quite different process from the one that was eventually described in published scientific papers. To see how that is so, and to better understand the nature of innovation in clinical medicine, we need to look in some detail at the language, style,
and structure of the paper by the Toronto group.

The researchers describe their study population with details about each baby
treated, including the birthweight, gestational age, complications of pregnancy or
delivery, mode of delivery, age at onset of IPPR, total hours on ventilation, and age
at death for those babies who died. They describe their techniques and methodologies with scientific precision:

> Following intubation and initiation of IPPR, a low tracheostomy was performed
> within 12 hours to facilitate the maintenance of a clear airway. All infants had serial
> arterial blood gas and chemical studies after admission, immediately before and after
> IPPR, and at 3- to 6-hour intervals for the first two days, then at 8- to 12-hour inter-
> vals. After the 6th day on the ventilator, blood and acid-base determinations were
> done daily. In 14 infants, the umbilical artery was catheterized with a No. 5 French
> polyvinyl tube filled with heparinized saline. On removal of the catheters blood was
> sampled by femoral artery puncture. All infants received 10% glucose intravenously
> (65 ml/kg/day) and sodium bicarbonate by slow syringe injection according to the es-
> timated base deficit. Blood transfusion was given (in 11 infants) in the presence of a
> hematocrit below 28%. Electrocardiogram, heart rate, respiratory rate, and colonic
> and environmental temperatures were monitored. Blood pH was measured by
> glass electrode, CO_2 content by means of Kopp-Natelson gasometer, PCO_2, by the
> Severinghaus electrode and PO_2s by the Clark electrode after a 15-minute period of
> breathing 100% O_2 on the ventilator. Plasma buffer base was derived from the Singer-
> Hastings nomogram. All measurements were made at 38 degrees C., and no correc-
> tion was made for the infant's body temperature.[8]

Such detail about the experimental conditions is a hallmark of good science. One wonders, however, whether such interventions as the daily acid-base determinations, the blood transfusions, or the umbilical artery catheterizations were actually part of the original study design or whether, in the process of innovating, the authors realized that these would be necessary and then, in the most forgivable sort of fictionalizing, described these innovations as if they were part of the study from the beginning. We do not know whether this is true, but it seems to be the only explanation for certain features of the protocol. Why, for example, did they start daily measurements of acid-base values only after day 6? Why did they pick a hematocrit of 28 percent as the threshold for blood transfusions? That no rationale is given for these seemingly arbitrary choices suggests, at the very least, an unconsidered process. It seems likely that the investigators were constantly innovating as they went along rather than implementing a set of predefined protocols.

They then report results that are cautiously optimistic, based on a criterion they did describe in their section on "Materials and Methods." In this result, they divide the babies into two groups—those who met eligibility criteria for IPPR in the first twenty-four hours of life and those who met eligibility criteria after twenty-four hours of life. All seven babies in the first group died after an average of seventy-two hours on the ventilator. Seven of thirteen babies in the second group survived. No baby who weighed less than 1800 grams at birth survived. From these findings, the authors conclude, "Our results suggest that if infants over 1800 g with failing respirations after 24 hours of age are placed on IPPR, and before a damaging degree of metabolic acidosis has developed, approximately one-half will survive with our present methods."[9]

Those results again raise as many questions as they resolve. The division into two groups seems to clearly be a post hoc analysis. That is, the researchers did not set out to test the hypothesis of whether early initiation of IPPR was superior to late initiation. They initiated IPPR and then noticed that it seemed to be working for some babies and not for others. They then report their results as if this was the hypothesis that they set out to test. They do this because they are enmeshed in the conceptual and linguistic model of clinical trials in which "methods" must precede "results." This model conveys the impression that researchers know what they are looking for before they find it. In fact, the opposite seems to be the case. Researchers often do not understand what questions to ask until they begin to gather and analyze data.

This process highlights a central theme of this book. It shows how the acquisition of knowledge in clinical medicine often follows a process that is conceptually quite different from the ideal model of clinical trial design. Investigators often do not develop hypotheses, design experiments to test them, analyze the results in ways that limit their inquiries to the hypotheses that they set out to test, and then use those results to develop new hypotheses. Instead, they innovate, retrospectively analyze the results of those innovations, and use those analyses to develop new innovations that they then evaluate in a similar way. It is experimental leapfrogging, rather than a sequential process of hypothesis development and testing.

This process is both messier and more fertile than the classic hypothesis-testing experiment. When a single hypothesis is being tested, the results are linear and straightforward and fairly unambiguous. The hypothesis is shown to be either compatible or incompatible with the results, to a certain degree of certainty. When, instead, innovation, data collection, post hoc analyses of data, and the generation of new hypotheses are performed simultaneously, any number of conclusions can be drawn. Different analysts will come up with alternative analyses of the same data. There is more room for speculation, creativity, and nuance as well as for error, mis interpretation, and diversions after false leads. It is a less orderly process but perhaps a more creative one.

So, for example, with the Toronto data on IPPR, one mystery in the way that the results are analyzed and reported is that the babies seemed to divide neatly into the two groups. The babies in the first group were all started on IPPR within 4–8 hours of birth, while the age at initiation for those in the second group ranged from 27 to 50 hours of age. Were there no babies who met eligibility criteria at 10 or 12 or 20 hours of age? Was this a physiological phenomenon, suggesting two very different disease processes, one with very early onset and one with much later onset? If so, then future treatment of the early onset group might require different considerations than treatment of the later onset group. Or was this, again, a deliberate choice of the researchers but one that, in this case, is not so carefully described—a choice borne, perhaps, of their early unsuccessful treatments?

The authors do not talk about what "failure" means. That is, they do not talk about what went into the decision to discontinue mechanical ventilation. Many babies were started on IPPR and then IPPR was stopped. In some cases, it was not restarted when the babies got worse. In other cases, however, it was restarted. Some babies went on and off the ventilators multiple times. How did the researchers decide whom to "reventilate" and whom to let die? Were these decisions, like the initial eligibility decisions, based on clinical criteria that were "obvious"? Again, the algorithms for making these decisions are not spelled out in the published paper.

The closest these authors come to an "ethical" assessment of what they are doing is in the comment that, for babies in group 1, the early-onset group, IPPR "merely prolongs, rather than saves, life." This cryptic comment has embedded within it a whole range of meanings that would be unpacked and explored over the next several decades. It might be thought of as the counterpart to the "eligibility criteria" by which babies were selected for participation in the innovative clinical trial. Eligibility criteria define the starting point of a trial. At the other end, we find the problem of "end points," markers by which clinical researchers might say that enough has been learned to determine whether the innovative treatment should be continued or withdrawn. These judgments require prognostic ability and a willingness to determine that further treatment is unlikely to be beneficial.

After reporting the methods and results of their study, the authors offer some political (or economic) opinions about the implications of their findings. They note that such treatment requires much more intensive monitoring by doctors and nurses than any treatment that had previously been given to newborns. For such interventions to be successful, they suggest that, "this method is completely dependent on continuous well-trained, experienced nursing and medical supervision, with 24-hour facilities for biochemical determinations. Infants undergoing assisted ventilation must never be left alone. Maintenance of adequate airflow into the lungs is crucial, and a breakdown of less than 5 minutes will reduce an infant in relatively good condition to a moribund state. For any hope of success, a suitable organization for intensive care incorporating the above principles is essential. We suggest that assisted ventilation should only be considered in centres where special facilities can be concentrated."[10]

With this comment, they clearly recognized that what they were proposing here was not a treatment that could be successfully used by doctors working in the clinical environments that existed at the time for the care of newborns. Instead, their innovation required, for its success, the creation of a vast new infrastructure—both to care for the babies who were receiving the IPPR treatment adequately but also and, perhaps, more importantly, to get those babies transferred to appropriate centers in a timely manner. This was not a scientific problem to be solved by more studies. It was a political and economic one to be solved by lobbying for alternative methods of resource allocation.

Interestingly, the parents are not mentioned in this paper. There is no discussion of whether informed consent was obtained, and no suggestion of whether some babies who were eligible for this innovative treatment did not receive it for any reason. This, too, is emblematic of the early days of neonatal research. Like the embedded controversies about the futility of standard treatments, the design of studies, the construction of eligibility criteria, and the validity of post hoc analyses, such omissions would be a central and problematic element of neonatal research.

Debates continue to this day about the proper role for parents, especially in the wide gray zone between standard interventions that are seen as ethically obligatory and innovative interventions that are seen as ethically optional.

This early paper on innovative use of positive pressure ventilation, then, has embedded within it all of the controversies that would swirl around neonatal intensive care for the next forty years. Which babies should be eligible for innovative therapies? Are there babies for whom treatment merely prolongs life, rather than saves it? How should the delivery of such services be organized (and who should pay)? To what extent were parents involved in the decisions about their babies?

The methodological problems that would haunt neonatal research in years to come are all there, too. This is not a randomized controlled trial. Instead, it relies entirely on historical controls. Would some babies who received mechanical ventilation have survived even without it? Were there some babies in the treatment group who were harmed by the treatment? It is impossible to tell from such a study.

Furthermore, this study presents just one method of treating the respiratory failure associated with hyaline membrane disease. At the same time, there were many other methods being developed, some as alternatives, some as complementary, all as potential parts of the developing algorithms of treatment that might be offered to different babies in different circumstances.

Cooke and colleagues in Copenhagen[11] and Reid and Tunstall's group in Aberdeen[12] reported long-term positive-pressure ventilation using nasotracheal intubation. This technique allowed maintenance of an artificial airway without the need for a tracheostomy (as used in the Toronto study), but it required new sorts of endotracheal tubes, clinical skill at intubation, new techniques to secure the tubes in place, and an even more rigorous need for continuous careful monitoring. These investigators raised concerns about the long-term complications associated with prolonged intubation and ventilation.[13] Previous reports had suggested laryngeal damage and subglottic stenosis as possible complications. Cooke and colleagues report one case of "laryngeal ulceration." Tunstall's group reports no such cases, and self-congratulatorily attributes their good outcomes to "scrupulous attention to detail" in managing their intubated patients.

Fear of the complications of long-term intubation and the recognition that intubation was less effective for the smallest babies than for larger babies led some investigators to try a whole different approach to the treatment of respiratory distress in newborns. In 1971, Gregory and colleagues in San Francisco reported their results using continuous positive airway pressure, or CPAP, to treat newborns with idiopathic respiratory distress syndrome (IRDS). They initiated the treatment on infants who were deteriorating on bag and mask ventilation. Unlike previous reports, Gregory's paper describes not just the babies who were in the study, but all of the babies admitted to their unit who were experiencing respiratory distress. They then describe their decision-making algorithm, explaining to readers how they chose babies for treatment or nontreatment. Over the sixteen-month period of the study, they treated fifty-one infants "who had classic clinical and roentgenographic evidence of IRDS."[14] Twenty-five of the fifty-one (49%) required only environmental oxygen or assisted ventilation with bag and mask. All survived. Twenty infants were unable to maintain a PaO_2 of greater than 50 mm of mercury while breathing 100 percent oxygen or had repeated episodes of apnea, cyanosis, or bradycardia. These infants were treated with CPAP and 16/20 (80%) survived. "Five infants were apneic at birth, never made spontaneous respiratory efforts, and therefore could not be treated with CPAP. Three were treated with IPPB and two with CPPB from birth. All died."[15]

Of the sixteen CPAP survivors, seven were under 1500 grams, suggesting that this technique might be better for tiny babies than the mechanical ventilation then being used in Toronto and other places. However, as the authors note, "comparisons between the survival of patients with IRDS treated with CPAP and other forms of therapy are difficult because each investigator has used different criteria for instituting assisted ventilation." They do note, however, that "regardless of the criteria used, survival in all series has been poor among infants weighing less than 1500g at birth or requiring assisted ventilation in the first 24 hours of life. In our group of 20 infants, 7 of 10 weighing less than 1500g survived, and 14 of 18 requiring assisted ventilation before 24 hours of age, survived."[16]

This study of CPAP, like the other studies of treatments for respiratory distress syndrome in newborns, was not a randomized trial. In this one, as in the others, there is no mention of the parents or their role and no discussion of whether this was considered "experimental" treatment or "research." There is a only cursory long-term follow-up:

> At the time of discharge from the hospital, no surviving infant had noteworthy hypoxemia or hypercarbia while breathing room air. The 16 survivors are now six to 18 months of age. Two have had two or three infections of the upper respiratory tract. One has had viral pneumonia, and one bronchitis; six have intercostal or subcostal retractions, and three have residual roentgenographic abnormalities. None are cyanotic. One infant is retarded in physical growth and neurologic development and has hydrocephalus due to a Dandy-Walker malformation. In the other infants, physical and neurologic development is normal if age is calculated from the date of conception.[17]

This description of long-term follow-up is as interesting for what it leaves out as for what it includes. Some of the children clearly have ongoing pulmonary disease, as evidenced by the roentgenographic and clinical findings. However, no blood gases or pulmonary function tests are described. The neurological and developmental outcomes are reported as "normal," although there is no description of the type of assessments on which that claim is based. In short, these follow-up data suggest more an awareness of concern about long-term outcomes than a serious attempt to quantify those outcomes.

Two years after this report, an editorial by Chernick in the journal *Pediatrics* discusses the difficulties in assessing the different techniques that are being used to treat respiratory disease in the newborn, the different studies that are being reported, and the rapid changes that are overtaking the field of newborn medicine. Chernick writes, "It is noteworthy that all of the published reports . . . to date have been noncontrolled studies. Proponents of these approaches to therapy were too much impressed with their results to attempt a controlled trial."[18] However, he seems more concerned with the aesthetics of this than with the science.

In this editorial, Chernick is raising another question that would follow neonatology through its development over the next several decades. How do we know that we know enough to stop studying something and start applying it? When do the interventions of neonatology stop being experimental and become standard therapy, stop being a hazard that babies must be shielded from, and start being a moral entitlement that must be provided to all babies?

THE DEVELOPMENT OF TOTAL PARENTERAL NUTRITION

The second key innovation of the late 1960s that transformed the treatment of premature babies was the development of TPN. The development of TPN differed from that of mechanical ventilation in a number of ways. First, mechanical ventilation had been used successfully in other clinical circumstances before it was applied to premature babies. Total parenteral nutrition, by contrast, had never been successfully used in other populations. In the 1960s, many doctors thought that it would be impossible to provide complete nutrition for any patient intravenously. In a recent historical review, Dudrick, a pioneer of TPN, wrote, "The prevailing dogma among clinicians in the 1960s was that feeding a patient entirely by vein was impossible. Even if it were possible, it would be impractical; even if it were practical, it would be unaffordable. Indeed, TPN was considered a 'Gordian knot' or a 'Holy Grail' pursuit by most physicians and surgeons."[19]

Second, TPN was developed primarily by surgeons rather than by pediatricians. Many of the earliest reports were in surgical journals. The goal of the treatment was initially to treat babies with complications of surgery, particularly the surgery that led to the "short-gut" syndrome.

Third, although initially created for the rare situation of short-gut syndrome, TPN would eventually be used as a preventive and supportive treatment for all premature babies rather than as an intervention to be used in life-threatening emergencies. Patients who need mechanical ventilation are generally suffering from life-threatening respiratory failure. Without treatment, death is imminent. Nutritional support, by contrast, is something that can lead to improvements in survival but not dramatically. It is a population-based, preventive treatment rather than an individualized crisis intervention. Each of these differences would be important in the way that TPN developed.

Most of the research that led to the successful clinical use of TPN took place at the University of Pennsylvania. Researchers there developed the precise combinations of chemicals to be infused and the techniques for infusing the TPN in laboratory experiments using dogs. Once these animal studies showed that the technology was feasible, they considered making the jump from animals to humans. As with mechanical ventilation, they had to decide who should go first—a choice in which they tried to balance the unknown risks of treatment with the known risks of nontreatment.

One of the first human patients to be given TPN was a newborn baby whose bowel had been surgically removed. Dudrick describes the case as follows:

> After massive intestinal resection, her duodenum had been anastomosed to the terminal 3 cm of ileum; her weight had declined from 2.5 kg at birth to 1.8 kg at 19 days of age; she appeared catabolic, hypometabolic, and moribund, and it was obvious that she was dying of starvation. After extensive consideration of the medical, moral, and ethical aspects of her problems, an *ad hoc* diverse committee of lay and professional people discussed, pondered, and debated every conceivable aspect of the proposed monumental and unprecedented experimental undertaking and were in accord that the risks of attempting to provide TPN by means of a central venous catheter in this infant were justifiable as the only reasonable option to save her life.[20]

This description of the process contains many of the same fundamental features as the descriptions of the early trials of IPPR; that is, the clinical assessment that the patient was dying, a risk-benefit assessment that TPN was as likely to help as to harm, cognizance of the ethical as well as the clinical issues, and, ultimately, a decision to venture into unknown clinical territory.

The infant almost immediately began to gain weight and to emerge from her moribund state, leading the investigators to conclude that the TPN treatment was successful. Although the baby was never able to eat by mouth, she was fed by vein for twenty-two months. Then she died.

Another similarity between this early trial of TPN and the early trials of IPPR is that it raised questions about varying notions of success. One wonders what the parents went through. They had a baby who otherwise would have died in infancy but who, as a result of their consent to an experimental intervention, lived for almost two years in the hospital and then died. Would they have chosen such an intervention again? We do not know because, in these reports, as in the IPPR reports, there is no mention of the parents' role in the decision-making process.

The success with this infant encouraged the Pennsylvania group to offer similar treatment to other infants. In 1969, they reported the results of such treatment in eighteen babies. It is a curious paper. In the "Methods and Materials" section, the authors say that "eighteen neonates with congenital anomalies of the gastrointestinal tract were supported by total parenteral nutrition for 7 to 400 days." In the "Results" section of the paper, they present a table that lists the results of the first twelve patients. The only "results" that they offer are the length of therapy (range 7–400 days, mean 59 days). They also include three "case reports," all of which seemed to have good outcomes. Two of the infants are described as having been discharged from the hospital, the third is reported to be gaining weight. Based on these results, they conclude that "few complications occurred in the use of total parenteral nutrition."[21]

These results in full-term neonates suffering from surgical complications were of enormous interest to neonatologists whose techniques of mechanical ventilation were now making it possible to keep tiny premature babies alive. Neonatology groups around the world began to use TPN clinically, often with very little careful study. By 1975, Winters, a pioneer of TPN, would report that "at present, there are clear definitions of indications and expectations of results for this method of therapy in two well-defined groups of patients—i.e., selected surgical neonates and infants with chronic intractable diarrhea. In addition, we have suggestive evidence of another potentially valuable application in the nutritional management of very low birthweight infants. However, in this group, a controlled study will be necessary before the role of total parenteral nutrition (TPN) in neonatal care of such infants can be determined precisely."[22]

Despite Winters's exhortation, TPN, like mechanical ventilation, diffused into clinical practice largely without any formal randomized trials. Instead, there was a steady stream of innovation, of case reports, of papers describing the particular practices of particular NICUs, their eligibility criteria, the particular infusates that they preferred, and the good and bad outcomes they observed. There was wide-spread practice variation. As with mechanical ventilation, the earliest innovators clearly recognized that the innovations they were developing had significant moral and economic implications. Their attempts to deal with these issues were as interesting and innovative as their attempts to develop new medical treatments. We will turn to those in the next section.

This detailed reading of the early reports of two clinical innovations in neonatology suggests a way of viewing medical progress that is somewhat at odds with conventional accounts. Instead of the careful testing of hypotheses through prospectively designed studies, there is wild and almost random innovation in particular centers where an atmosphere of innovative exuberance has taken hold. At some such centers, the innovations were carefully studied and the data were taken apart, reformulated, and scrutinized. Results are observed, documented, analyzed, and reported to peers. There was openness to inquiry about what worked and what did not. Part of the process involved the tentative formation of hypotheses but often the hypotheses did not become the foundation of a formal, well-designed clinical trial. Instead, they become the basis for a series of further innovative changes that created the possibility of future inquiries. At other centers, no such studies were carried out. Instead, practices were institutionalized immediately into rigid dogma.

There was an ongoing debate between the proponents of more formal clinical trials for every innovation and those who thought that the rigid format of clinical trials would inhibit progress rather than validate it. In some ways, the debate was misleading. Formal clinical trials took on a totemic quality, as if they alone could reify practice into knowledge. A more nuanced view was expressed in an editorial about early trials of mechanical ventilation. "One or two controlled studies of the use of distending pressure in severe hyaline membrane disease, although daring, are welcome; many more would be foolish. Since this method of therapy has been clearly proved to increase arterial Po_2, the potential risk of *not* treating infants by its use is too great to be denied, despite the fact that we cannot predict at the present time which infants will ultimately succumb to a complication."[23]

MORAL ISSUES OF NEONATAL INTENSIVE CARE
IN THE 1960s and 1970s

The evolution of ethical analysis about the issues of neonatal intensive care was quite analogous to the evolution of scientific knowledge. In the beginning, people did not really understand how to articulate or analyze the real and important ethical issues they sensed. Instead, these conundrums were vaguely perceived by a few intuitive and far-seeing souls, just as the possibility of clinical innovation could sometimes be perceived in advance. At some professional meetings, the doctors who were inventing neonatology took the seemingly bizarre and, at that time, unprecedented step of inviting philosophers and theologians to speculate about and help wrestle with the ethical issues. As these morally troubled doctors worked with the philosophers to articulate their concerns, they came to propose moral analyses that might apply to the tough decisions faced by doctors and parents. These forays into the development of moral theory were as tentative, as innovative, and perhaps even as "experimental" as the clinical interventions themselves. These were, after all, moral problems of an entirely new breed. Philosophers were in the same position as the clinical investigators—vaguely aware of both the potential benefits of such treatment approaches as well as the potential dangers—but were initially unable to define precisely or categorize correctly the moral categories into which choices among them might belong. As a result, the understanding of the ethical issues and of the appropriate responses to them evolved just as the clinical innovations evolved.

The roots of future moral conflicts were inherent in the innovative technologies. Even in the earliest days of neonatology, innovators understood that the tension at the very center of the project in which they were engaged was the tension between the potential of techniques that they were developing to save the lives of previously doomed premature babies and the possibility that those techniques would be only partially effective, saving life but not curing the diseases to which premature babies were heirs. In theological terms, the blessings of neonatology might be so tainted with curses that it would be hubris to seek them.

As early as 1968, pioneering neonatologist Jerold Lucey convened a conference of leading innovators to consider where the young field was heading. In his introductory remarks to the conference, he described how many hospitals had already created special care nurseries "in an effort to reduce neonatal mortality and hopefully to increase the number of intellectually intact survivors." He acknowledged that problems and controversies existed because "it is too early to judge the overall effectiveness of these efforts."[24] The conference was a first attempt to make an assessment of these problems and controversies.

The conference was not focused on ethics per se. However, it soon became apparent that there were ethical issues inextricably intertwined with the clinical issues. When speakers tried to assess the efficacy of neonatal intensive care and examined both the overall survival rates and what they called "intact survival"— without any data or what "intact" actually meant—they were tiptoeing toward controversies that were more complex than they imagined. At that early point in the development of the specialty, there did not seem to be much awareness that there would be deep disagreements about the implications of judgments that some babies were not intact enough to be given life-sustaining treatment. Instead, they were concerned that they would be criticized for saving babies whose "non-intact-ness" would undermine support for the entire specialty.

Mildred Stahlman of Vanderbilt University, a neonatologist who attended the conference put it like this, "One must conclude that we have probably preserved some of those infants' lives only to have them survive with cerebral palsy, mental retardation, or both. For this we must assume responsibility, as well as for those bright attractive children who were in a respirator for hyaline membrane disease."[25] In more blunt terms, she seemed to be saying that if too many premature babies survived with neurologic deficits, the field would be judged a failure.

Dr. Stahlman argued that, on the whole, neonatology should be judged a success for three reasons. First, she demonstrated that there had been significant improvements in birthweight-specific survival rates. Second, she showed that many of the survivors who accounted for these improvements were neurologically intact. Finally, she argued that overall rates of "non-intact" survival had not changed; instead, there was a shift in the subpopulations of babies with different outcomes— that babies who might have survived with deficits before the introduction of neonatal intensive care were now surviving intact but that some babies who otherwise would have died were now surviving with neurological problems. Thus, she did not see neonatal intensive care as increasing overall rates of cerebral palsy, mental retardation, or blindness. Instead, she saw it as creating choices and responsibilities in situations where heretofore there had been only fate, an argument that would become familiar over time and one for which the data are mixed, confusing, and inconclusive.

The 1968 Lucey conference had not focused on ethics, but it raised so many thorny issues that some participants were eager to meet again to focus specifically on ethical concerns. Four years later, Stahlman hosted a meeting entitled, "Ethical Dilemmas in Current Obstetric and Newborn Care." Stahlman began by alluding to Gertrude Stein, hoping that even if the conference could not answer all the questions it might at least frame them well. Dr. Wolf Zuelzer framed the ethical dilemmas of newborn care as follows, "How can we go about implementing a policy of judicious neglect, assuming that a consensus of principle exists or can be generated? Who is to make the decisions that would deprive a human, however defective, of a chance to live? What criteria in terms of medical, genetic, sociological, and psychological knowledge shall we use? What safeguards would be required to protect us against a Hitlerian type of eugenics?"[26]

Two philosophers, Joseph Fletcher and Robert Veatch, were present at this conference. Fletcher was 67 years old and nearing the end of a career as a theologian and medical ethicist. Veatch, at age 33, was near the beginning of his career. Fletcher's background was in Episcopal theology. Veatch was initially trained as a pharmacologist but went on to do graduate studies in philosophy. The two philosophers articulated very different approaches to the dilemmas of the NICU.

Fletcher argued for a principle-based utilitarian consistency by which the end might justify the means. In discussing those babies whom he called "defective newborns," he described four options. "One, to kill them; two, to starve them; three, just not help them; four, to treat and preserve them." Then he asked, "Are not the first three in that list actually gradations of the same thing? Morally speaking, is there really any difference? I would contend they are the same thing. The end sought is the same: the infant's death." From this starting point, he argued that the fundamental decision to be made was whether the life of the infant was worth preserving. If not, and if, as he thought, options one through three were morally equivalent, then practitioners in the field should have the moral courage to both acknowledge this and to act on it.[27]

This approach is interesting for its abstract philosophic rigor. It is, on its own terms, powerful and internally consistent, the sort of reasoning that many philosophers (and some lawyers) would use to argue that there was no distinction between, on the one hand, withholding or withdrawing of life-sustaining treatment and, on the other hand, the active administration of a lethal drug. Such arguments were most coherently elucidated by philosopher James Rachels in a 1975 paper on the similarities or differences between killing and letting die. Rachels argued that, because so-called active euthanasia was morally indistinguishable from so-called passive euthanasia, it followed, logically, that any situation in which it was morally permissible to withdraw life support became also a situation in which it was morally permissible to give a lethal injection. Rachels further argued that, because the two actions were morally equivalent, there may be situations in which active euthanasia was preferable because it was more painless. Fletcher was echoing these arguments in his opinions about the treatment, nontreatment, or deliberate euthanizing of newborns.

Veatch's position was less forthright but was a clear challenge to Fletcher. He argued less about the substantive criteria that might be used to determine which infants' lives were worth preserving and more about the procedural criteria that might be used to determine who should be empowered to make decisions about such babies. He made a claim that was quite radical at the time, suggesting that it was parents, not doctors, who should have the right to make decisions, "even if that course of action includes exercising the right to receive treatment" that doctors (or philosophers) might not recommend. He expressed "shock and outrage" at the physicians and philosophers who argued that they alone knew what was best for babies with congenital anomalies. In shifting the focus thus from the abstract moral principles that might justify or prohibit a given action to the process of decision making and the locus of moral authority, Veatch heralded the change in focus of the bioethics movement in such cases over the next decades. Doctor-driven principalism would give way to patient-driven proceduralism, at least with regard to decisions about end of life care.

Pediatric surgeon Judson Randolph challenged Veatch, asking him, "Doctor Veatch, why are you shocked and angered?" Veatch replied, "Physicians continue to assume that they have the right, even the duty, to benevolently make decisions for patients. Many laymen are taking this as an assault on their dignity as humans and their right to control decisions which affect their own bodies."

In framing the issues this way, Fletcher and Veatch presaged the debates that would occur over the next two decades. Doctors were caught between the prevailing paradigms, uncertain if they were obligated to exercise their own values, to reflect societal values, or to ascertain the parents' values. From the 1970s until now, these three loci of moral authority would remain important and in tension. The general trend over that time period would be a gradual shift from the sort of doctor-driven moral hierarchy that Randolph understood and advocated to the sort of parent-driven hierarchy Veatch championed.

These issues would be taken up again a few years later at a conference in Sonoma, California, where experts tried to develop a set of guidelines for neonatology. The conferees began by noting that "most medical interventions effect some harm, either transient or permanent; that harm is usually justified by an expected compensatory benefit. If no benefit can be reasonably expected or if the benefit does not compensate for the harm, the intervention is unethical. The assessment of whether the benefit does compensate for the harm lies principally with the patient, who must suffer the harm. In the case of infants, the assessment must be made by those who bear responsibility and duty within a context of broad social understanding."[28] They then tried to articulate guidelines for situations in which it might be considered appropriate to discontinue life-sustaining treatment. Their summary sentence was, "In the context of certain irremediable life conditions, intensive care therapy appears harmful. These conditions are . . . [the] inability to survive infancy, inability to live without severe pain, and inability to participate, at least minimally, in human experience."[29]

This concise statement summarizing the moral rationale for allowing a baby to die rather than continuing potentially life-sustaining treatment has been a touchstone for every clinical ethics judgment made ever since. It is as much a fundamental discovery as, say, the discovery that premature babies lack pulmonary surfactant. And it has been generative in the same way. That is, the discovery itself was fundamental, but the implications of the discovery would take decades to work out, would lead to unanticipated controversies, and would eventually transform the field. In both cases, the basic discovery has not been questioned or seriously challenged. Instead, it has led to attempts to take the discovery from theory to practice, from bench to bedside.

In these early papers and conferences about the ethics of newborn care, the tensions were clear. There were disputes about abstract philosophical principles. The law was also a factor. Every baby had both legal rights that could be defended in court and moral rights that could be defended in theory. The parents also had some legal rights. Legally, they had the right to make medical decisions for their baby unless that right was taken away by a court that found them neglectful. But parents also had responsibilities. They were obligated to make decisions based on the interests of the baby. In some cases, the parents' desires conflicted with what seemed to be the baby's interests. Doctors were then torn between their desire to do what was best for the baby and their desire to respect the parents' rights. The state, through the courts, had the role of protecting the interests of vulnerable citizens, and often, though not always, deferred to medical judgments to define those interests.

As the scientific studies were proceeding, questions about resolving these conflicting rights and responsibilities arose. They were made more urgent because of the economic and administrative issues raised by the new therapies. Before the 1960s, care of newborns had not been highly technical, highly expensive, or particularly successful. As a result, questions about what we, collectively, owed to babies were more theoretical than practical. Mechanical ventilation and TPN changed all that. New administrative and political solutions became necessary to distribute the goods of this scientific and technological breakthrough. Those solutions, in turn, transformed the landscape of moral decision making in fundamental ways.

THE DEVELOPMENT OF REGIONALIZATION

As early as 1970, leaders of neonatology were advocating for the creation of regionalized networks for perinatal care. Given the decentralized nature of the health care system in the United States, the likelihood of implementing a comprehensive system of regionalization seemed small. It would require a number of unprecedented political rearrangements. First, because regionalization in this domain would require centers that could care for both pregnant women and their newborns, it would require a new level of cooperation between obstetricians and pediatricians. Second, regionalization would require complex and cooperative interrelationships between community hospitals and centralized referral centers. Finally, because tertiary care NICUs could only be created with an initial outlay of capital, regionalization would require new and innovative funding mechanisms.

Leaders of the field conceptualized the scope of this transformation by arguing that "this area of medical care is so different from others that it can be administered satisfactorily only by specially trained people working within an organization specifically designed and equipped for the purpose."[30] In other words, they envisioned the creation of a separate administrative zone within medicine, governed by different people and different rules than those which prevailed in other zones of medicine.

The articulation of such a vision required bold leadership. The implementation of it suggests just how unique neonatal intensive care was in the 1970s. After all, medical leaders in many other subspecialties had long recognized the potential advantages of regionalized systems of care. Studies showed that regionalization could lower costs and improve quality. On the basis of such studies, most other countries developed regionalized systems that improved quality and lowered cost. In the United States, regionalization was advocated for cardiac care,[31] for major surgical procedures,[32] and for the health system as a whole.[33] In the 1970s, federal laws were passed to try to create regional authorities that would rationalize the allocation of resources, avoid the unnecessary duplication of costly technology, and concentrate expertise in referral centers. However, few such systems were actually implemented.

Perinatal care was the interesting exception. There were three reasons why perinatal regionalization was possible. First, there was unique professional leadership from many different medical specialties. Second, the economics of neonatal care were such that it was unclear whether such programs would be profitable or costly to hospitals. As a result, hospitals were less entrepreneurial in this area than they were in areas of medicine where the economics of profitability were more straightforward. Finally, because babies were not Medicare beneficiaries, there was no need to develop a single national program. The requirement to do so often led to disagreements based on regional preferences. In neonatal care, by contrast, different states could develop their own unique regionalized programs that were more sensitive to local needs.

Professional leadership began early with an explicit and well-planned lobbying campaign within organized medicine. L. Joseph Butterfield, the director of the Newborn Center of the Children's Hospital of Denver introduced the concept of regionalization to the AMA Committee on Maternal and Child Care at their meeting in Chicago in 1970. The AMA Committee formed a subcommittee charged with developing a policy statement to present to the AMA's Board of Trustees and House of Delegates. In a review of those events, Butterfield writes, "After review and endorsement by the AMA Board of Trustees, the policy statement was considered by the AMA House of Delegates in August of 1971 and adopted as AMA policy! This was a landmark day in American medicine and a futuristic statement on perinatal medicine by the AMA."[34] The policy was then endorsed by the American Academy of Pediatrics, the American Academy of Family Physicians, and the American College of Obstetrics and Gynecology. This was an unprecedented endorsement of regionalized planning by leaders of organized medicine in the United States. But it was only the first step.

The next step was to develop detailed guidelines for regionalized programs. The challenge was to come up with guidelines that were substantive but flexible. The process of coming up with guidelines takes work and work costs money. A key alliance was formed between leaders in pediatrics, obstetrics, and the National Foundation / March of Dimes. The March of Dimes, originally founded to fund research about polio, had shifted the focus of its philanthropy to the problem of neonatal mortality. The organization endorsed the regionalization of perinatal services as an important step toward improving neonatal outcomes and gave funding for a planning process. With funding from the March of Dimes, the AAP, AMA, ACOG, and AAFP created a Committee on Perinatal Health that formed task forces to write a detailed report on the mechanisms to institute, finance, and monitor regionalized perinatal networks. That report, published in 1976, became the basis for many states' regionalized programs.

This work of these visionary professional leaders set the stage, then, for the tougher challenge of solving the complex political and economic problems faced by hospitals and practitioners who would each need to decide whether to support the development of regionalized programs and, more importantly, participate in them. Both hospitals and practitioners in the United States are generally suspicious about the monopolistic aspects of regionalized programs. After all, the whole goal of such programs is to create a single center that captures all of the business in one particular area of medicine. In doing so, regionalized programs not only achieve the goals for which they were designed—improving quality and lowering costs— but they also garner all of the excitement and prestige that goes along with the provision of "cutting edge" medical services. Every tertiary care hospital wants to be a leader in this regard. Few voluntarily agree to defer to their competitors. Every doctor wants to practice in a hospital that provides all such services. Implementation and sustenance of any regionalized program, therefore, depends upon balancing complex economic and psychological incentives that motivate many different individuals and institutions.

For the development of regional neonatal programs, hospitals were the key stakeholder. This is because NICUs required, first and foremost, a significant capital investment in both technology and personnel. Hospitals, even allegedly not-for-profit hospitals, generally support programs that bring in revenue. If NICUs were clearly going to be unprofitable, few hospitals would have wanted to create them and there would have been no tertiary care centers. If NICUs were clearly going to be profitable, every hospital would have wanted one. Part of what made regionalization possible in the 1970s was the fact that the economic incentives were ambiguous. It was unclear whether the tertiary care centers would make money or lose money by developing high-risk obstetric services and NICUs that would accept the transfers of high-risk mothers and babies.

The development of regionalization in the state of Illinois offers an interesting case study of how these various forces played out. The state passed legislation to implement a regionalized perinatal program in the mid-1970s. Under the legislation, the state decided how many tertiary care centers they needed, and hospitals could then opt in or opt out. Hospital administrators had to decide, then, whether they wanted to participate in the statewide program by becoming a perinatal referral center. Most hospitals in Illinois were not among the pioneering hospitals in neonatology. Many had no NICUs at all. So the hospital administrators and doctors faced an interesting dilemma. They had to decide whether to bet on the future of neonatology as a medical enterprise and as an economic one. A decision not to participate might save money but might also leave them out of an important and growing area of modern medicine. A decision to participate might enmesh them in a dense new web of government regulation that would chain them to what might turn out to be a money-losing proposition.

The University of Chicago Hospital was typical in its response to this dilemma. It is located in a poor neighborhood on the south side of the city. Many of the patients in the university's catchment area had no insurance or were insured by Medicaid. The prospects for profitability in neonatal care were not good. The infrastructure necessary to become a perinatal center would require a significant up-front investment. There was no champion among the pediatricians on the medical staff.

Hospital administrators initially cautioned against providing such services. Then Dr. Jack Madden, a pediatrician, stepped forward who, interestingly, had not previously been particularly interested in the emerging science of neonatology. Instead, Dr. Madden was a primary care pediatrician who had spent most of the 1960s working in a community health center providing preventive care services to poor mothers and children. He recognized, however, that the political support for preventive care services and community health centers, which had been strong in the 1960s, was eroding in the 1970s. By contrast, the support for regionalized NICUs seemed to be an area in which there was political support and through which the hospital might equally well serve the community on Chicago's poor south side.

Dr. Madden convinced the university's administrators to participate in the statewide perinatal regionalization program. They did so somewhat half-heartedly. The initial NICU at University of Chicago, like the NICUs in many hospitals, was poorly funded and had inadequate space. However, it had more resources than it might have had without the regionalization legislation that imposed regulations on any participating tertiary care center. Chicago's experience illustrates how the attentiveness to the particularities of each local medical, political and economic culture was crucial to the successful implementation of regionalization.

Part of the reason that perinatal regionalization was able to happen was because the two administrative entities that oversaw the care of poor mothers and children were the Medicaid program and the state health departments. One group of state health department officials described their motivations as follows, "The interest of state health departments in programs such as regionalization of perinatal care stems from concerns for the promotion of high-quality maternal and child health services, efficient utilization of health facility and health manpower resources, and the economical provision of health care."[35]

As with the hospitals, however, the involvement of state health departments was not without tensions. State health departments, traditionally, were much more concerned with public health than with hospital-based technologies. Neonatal intensive care, at the beginning, was an unusual amalgam of high-tech, tertiary care medicine and grass-roots public health medicine. The two zones of concern came together through their mutual focus upon lowering infant mortality. Before the advent of NICUs, most infant mortality programs were of the sort more traditionally associated with public health—population-based, low-tech, preventive treatments such as the provision of prenatal care or immunizations, or the encouragement of safe feeding practices.

One of the interesting political alliances that allowed neonatal regionalization was between those motivated primarily by a desire to develop and study innovative treatments in NICUs and those who were more generally motivated by a desire to lower infant mortality rates by any effective means. State public health departments generally fell into the latter group. Because they administered Medicaid programs, and because so many premature babies were insured by Medicaid, the health departments had unique fiscal leverage over the tertiary care hospitals in this area. As Ann Pettigrew, health commissioner of Massachusetts, wrote, "Many state health departments are also empowered to develop standards or conditions of participation for a variety of State and Federal programs, such as Medicaid and Crippled Children's Programs. Noncompliance with these standards can mean decertification and denial of reimbursement funds under that particular program."[36]

The development of regionalization in Massachusetts was typical of such developments throughout the country. The State Health Department created a task force with all stakeholders at the table. The task force began by establishing specific definitions and requirements for special care nurseries, including precise staffing requirements and descriptions of the appropriate qualifications and training for staff working the neonatal units. These guidelines and definitions were then used, as they were in Illinois, to cajole hospitals to upgrade their services in order to become a designated regional referral center.

The flexibility afforded by the state-based locus of control was crucial because not all states were the same. In California, initiatives came not from state agencies but from hospital personnel. In Long Beach, California, for example, a hospital task force developed a plan to create a regionalized perinatal center that would serve two hospitals in the area. The challenge they faced was daunting. There were two hospitals in town that provided obstetrics services. The new regionalized center, if it was to be effective, would have to be at one or the other. They solved this problem by creating a Perinatal Center that was administratively separate from each of the hospitals, though it was located at one of them. The Perinatal Center had a separate Board of Trustees and offered its own medical staff privileges, though the doctors also had staff privileges at one or the other hospital. In describing this solution, one of the leaders noted, "The concept of a separate medical staff and advisory Board of Trustees, layered over an existing organization structure, may not fit traditional concepts and might actually be frightening to students of organization theory. However the concept has worked effectively."[37]

These mini case studies from Illinois, Massachusetts and California suggest the complexity of the process in each city, state, or region. Eventually, these local and statewide efforts led to a somewhat comprehensive system of regionalized perinatal care that covered most of the United States. Hospitals were designated as level 1, level 2, or level 3, with level 1 being the least sophisticated and level 3 being the tertiary care referral centers. The goal of regionalization was to have all high-risk deliveries take place in a level 3 center. Success in reaching this goal varied by region. One easily measurable statistic in assessing success was the percentage of very low birthweight (VLBW) babies delivered in level 1 centers. By the 1990s, in California, 10.5 percent of all VLBW infants were delivered in level 1 hospitals. Significant variation across regions of the state was evident, ranging from a regional low of 3.1 percent to a high of 24.3 percent.[38] In Ohio, there was similar variation—a total of 59.8 percent of VLBW infants were born in a level 3 hospital, with significant regional variations among the six perinatal regions.[39] In South Carolina, 78 percent of VLBW deliveries occurred in level 3 hospitals.[40]

These statistics suggest that the development of regionalization in perinatal care was good but not perfect—different states were different, different regions within states were different, and the differences persisted over time. Nevertheless, in each state and region, the goal of maintaining regionalized networks was maintained. This made perinatal care one of the few areas of American medicine in which regionalized care was recognized as a goal, implemented broadly, and maintained.

LEGAL CASES IN THE 1970S

In the 1970s, the legal issues surrounding decisions to withhold or withdraw treatment from newborns were murky, unformed, and contradictory. Yet, there seemed to be widespread awareness that such decisions were common in nurseries all across America. After all, articles by leading pediatricians and pediatric surgeons in leading medical journals had described such decisions and had argued that they were appropriate in some circumstances.

In one article, Drs. Raymond Duff and Arthur Campbell, two pediatricians at Yale–New Haven Hospital, described the circumstances surrounding each of the 299 deaths that had occurred during the preceding thirty months in their special care nursery. Their report began in a fairly dry and statistical fashion. They noted that 299 (14%) of the 2171 infants who were admitted to the Yale special care nursery died. After analyzing the cases, they discovered that 256, or 86 percent, of these deaths occurred despite the babies' receiving every available treatment. That is, in most cases, there was no decision to withhold or withdraw life-sustaining treatment. Most of those deaths were in babies with extreme prematurity or respiratory problems. Their report then focused on the remaining forty-three deaths, the 14 percent of the total that were associated with decisions by doctors and parents to withhold or withdraw treatment. Fifteen of those babies had congenital anomalies such as myelomeningocele. Another eight of the forty-three had chromosomal abnormalities such as Down syndrome.

Duff and Campbell describe in great detail their conversations with parents about whether to continue treatment for critically ill babies. They report how every family was different. In some cases, they note, the doctors thought it would be appropriate to stop treatment and parents opted for continued treatment. In others, the parents requested the discontinuation of further therapy and the doctors acceded. They note that there were sometimes disagreements among the nursery staff about whether such decisions were the right. "Some contended that individuals should have a right to die in some circumstances such as anencephaly, hydranencephaly, and some severely deforming and incapacitating conditions . . . Others considered allowing a child to die wrong for several reasons." Duff and Campbell note that "some physicians recognized that the wishes of families went against their own, but they were resolute. They commonly agreed that if they were the parents of very defective children, withholding treatment would be most desirable for them. However, they argued that aggressive management was indicated for others."[41]

Duff and Campbell stayed in touch with parents in the months after the deaths. In their opinion, the "families appear to have experienced a normal mourning for their losses. Although some have exhibited doubts that the choices were correct, all appear to be as effective in their lives as they were before this experience."[42]

In the same issue of the New England Journal of Medicine, Dr. Anthony Shaw, a pediatric surgeon at the University of Virginia, raised questions about "rights and obligations of physicians, parents and society in situations in which parents withhold consent for treatment of their children."[43] Four of the eight cases that he described were of babies with Down syndrome and other anomalies whose parents refused to consent to life-saving surgery. Shaw reports that these babies were allowed to die.

Both articles conclude that parents and doctors should make such difficult decisions together. Duff and Campbell write, "We believe the burdens of decision making must be borne by families and their professional advisers because they are most familiar with the respective situations . . . We do not know how often families and their physicians will make just decisions for severely handicapped children. Clearly, this issue is central in evaluation of the process of decision making that we have described. But we also ask, if these parties cannot make such decisions justly, who can?" Similarly, Shaw concludes, "I think that the parents must participate in any decision about treatment and they must be fully informed of the consequences of consenting and of withholding treatment."[44] Both papers see these decisions as ones that do not require societal oversight. Duff and Campbell give a little more authority to parents. Shaw leans more toward the physicians. But neither foresaw the societal concerns that would dominate this debate. Neither, apparently, did the editors of the *New England Journal of Medicine*, who printed the articles without commentary.

Many theologians writing at the time held similar attitudes. Joseph Fletcher was one of the first theologians to become interested in medical ethics. In his book, *Situation Ethics,* he talks about such cases and advocates a mode of decision making that is sensitive to the nuances of the situation, rather than a mode that seeks to apply rigid rules in all situations. The net effect of his approach would be similar to the approach advocated by Shaw, Duff, and Campbell, namely, to empower the parents to make decisions based on their own personal, moral views.

Other theologians struggled with these issues and came to somewhat different conclusions. James Gustafson, another Protestant theologian, wrote in 1973 about a case at Johns Hopkins University Hospital that involved a baby with Down syndrome. Gustafson raises questions about the societal implications of such decisions and invites speculation on whether such decisions are, in fact, private. His conclusions are tentative. He writes, "To be sure, the parents are ambiguous about their feelings for a mongoloid infant, since it is normal to desire a normal infant rather than an abnormal infant. But once the infant is born, its independent existence provides independent value in itself, and those who brought it into being and those professionally responsible for its care have an obligation to sustain its life regardless of their negative or ambiguous feelings toward it . . . The only reasonable conclusion is that the surgery ought to have been done."[45]

Surveys of pediatricians showed that many had made decisions similar to those of Duff, Campbell, and Shaw or had approved such decisions.[46] There were even documentary movies about such decisions and scholarly papers analyzing those movies. Clearly, by the early 1970s, such decisions for newborns were much more public than similar decisions for adults.

By contrast, many legal scholars who analyzed the legal implications of these decisions concluded that there was no legal framework within which such decisions could be considered legally safe and no reason why doctors and parents could not be prosecuted. Robertson and Fost wrote in 1976, "There appears to be criminal liability on several grounds for parents, physicians, nurses, and administrators. Such liability may include charges of homicide by omission, child neglect, and failure to report child neglect. Increasing public exposure of the practice increases the probability that such prosecutions may be brought. Individuals involved in such decisions should be aware of their possible legal liability."[47]

As Ellis noted in a review published in 1982, "The literature discloses no reported case or decision imposing criminal liability for decisions not to treat seriously defective newborns. Both health professionals and the public have seriously misinterpreted this absence of judicial precedent. They have concluded that the absence of controlling judicial precedent means that the issue is 'open' and that parents and physicians are therefore free to proceed without fear of legal challenge or liability."[48] Ellis, like others who studied the issue carefully, concluded that applicable statutes concerning "homicide, manslaughter, and child neglect" were operative and applicable.

There seemed to be a mysterious disjunction between medical practice and legal theory in this area in the 1970s. It was not from lack of attention or awareness. Instead, it seemed to result from the recognition that things were changing. It led to a sincere struggle to figure out which of the potentially applicable legal paradigms to choose and a careful analysis of how they should be applied.

There were a number of potentially available legal paradigms. Decisions to withhold life-sustaining treatment might be considered homicide or manslaughter. After all, they were decisions taken with the foreknowledge that they would lead to the death of another person. Often the goal was to bring about the death of that person. Such actions seemed to meet all the legal criteria of homicide or manslaughter. The piece that seemed to be missing was the motive. Intuitively, if not legally, homicide or manslaughter was generally thought to require malice or at least negligence. In most cases involving newborns, the motives seemed to be different and more complex, a mixture of humanism, compassion, judgments about quality of life, and perhaps an intrafamilial utilitarianism by which parents were allowed or even encouraged to allocate their resources to some children even if it meant denying them to others.

Alternatively, such decisions might be considered instances of child abuse or medical neglect rather than homicide or manslaughter. The conceptual framework for this approach was the common-law notion that parents have a legal obligation to provide appropriate medical care for their children. Lifesaving interventions are generally considered appropriate, so the refusal to seek or to authorize lifesaving interventions might be considered a breach of this parental responsibility.

Society's approach to child abuse and neglect was changing dramatically in the 1970s. In 1974, Congress first passed legislation defining child abuse and providing modest funding for state child protection agencies.[49] Before that, child abuse had been seen as a local problem or, in some locales, a nonexistent problem. This legislation drew attention to the problem and allowed research to begin to quantify the prevalence of different forms of abuse, including physical, sexual, and emotional abuse as well as medical neglect.

A different rubric for analyzing the legal issues associated with nontreatment of newborns was as a form a discrimination against individuals with disabilities. After all, as one commentator noted, "virtually all children selected for non-treatment are obviously and extremely handicapped."[50] Like child abuse, however, the prevention of discrimination on the basis of disability was a relatively new legal concept. The federal law defining such discrimination as a violation of civil rights had been enacted only in 1973. The potentially relevant portion of that law stated, "No otherwise qualified handicapped individual in the United States . . . shall, solely by reason of his handicap, be excluded from participation in, be denied the benefits of, or be subjected to discrimination under any program or activity receiving federal financial assistance."[51] Because the law was so new, it was unclear whether it would apply to nontreatment decisions of newborns made on the basis of a disabling condition such as Down syndrome or spina bifida.

Another legal arena in which such issues might be resolved was the area of civil liability. As Ellis noted, "Parents might sue physicians and other health care providers for negligence, wrongful death, abandonment, or breach of an implied contract . . . Even where consent is obtained, questions may arise concerning the adequacy of information supplied to the parents or guardian."[52]

However, there were legal frameworks wherein decisions to withhold or withdraw life-sustaining treatment would have been considered legal, appropriate, ethical, and perhaps obligatory. During the 1970s, courts were struggling to define the legal issues surrounding the withholding of life support for adult patients. Some courts found that the constitutional right to privacy that had been articulated in cases of reproductive health might apply to these other medical decisions. Cases such as the one involving Karen Quinlan framed the issue in terms of a constitutional right to privacy and the right of a competent adult to refuse medical interventions. These could not be readily applied to children. Quality of life criteria were difficult to operationalize because, in the context of "wrongful birth" or "wrongful life" lawsuits, the courts generally held (following the New Jersey Supreme Court) that "one of the most deeply held beliefs in our society is that life—whether experienced with or without a major physical handicap—is more precious than non-life."[53]

It is interesting and mysterious that, during this time period, with its widespread awareness that decisions were being made to allow babies to die, and the widespread understanding that there was no applicable legal framework under which such decisions might be considered protected from criminal or civil liability, there were no criminal prosecutions. In fact, the cases that came to legal attention were generally cases in which there was disagreement among professionals or between professionals and parents about whether medical treatment ought to be considered mandatory. The courts, then, were not asked after the fact whether to punish people who made decisions to withhold or withdraw treatment. Instead, they were asked, before the fact, whether such treatment was legally mandatory or whether it could be forgone. Furthermore, the cases that came to court were cases where there was a conflict, and the conflict was generally between parents who did not want treatment and doctors who thought it should be provided.

In a Maine case in which a baby was born with multiple congenital anomalies, the parents wanted to let the baby die. The doctors petitioned the court to take protective custody and to order treatment that they believed to be in the baby's interest. The judge determined that the parents had no right to withhold life-sustaining treatment.[54] In a California case involving a child with Down syndrome and a surgically correctable heart defect, the child's parents rejected surgery. The staff of the group home where he lived disagreed. They petitioned the court, which ordered the surgery. The parents of a 3 year old with cancer in Massachusetts preferred laetrile to chemotherapy. The pediatric oncologist petitioned the court to order chemotherapy. The court agreed.[55] These cases set the judicial precedent for situations in which doctors thought treatment was appropriate and parents did not. There were no cases, however, where parents wanted treatment and doctors did not or where doctors and parents together decided to stop treatment. In the 1970s, the courts were more concerned about adjudicating disagreements than they were about creating new policies regarding nontreatment decisions. That would change in the following decades.

CHAPTER FOUR

The Era of Exposed Ignorance, 1982–1992

This decade saw widespread medical, political, and legal controversy following the death of a baby, Baby Doe in Bloomington, Indiana. Before telling that story, however, we review the medical developments that set the stage for the national controversy. Medical advances during the first era of neonatology were characterized by the development of two key therapeutic interventions: mechanical ventilation and TPN. We have argued that the development of these interventions took place in ways that did not reflect prevailing norms of epidemiology, epistemology, or ethics. The advances were not the result of well-designed randomized trials conducted with prior approval of a research ethics committee and with the informed consent of patients or parents. Instead, they were the result of exuberant innovation by enthusiastic investigators who brought together their own clinical insights, the results of animal research, scientific theory, and a moral zeal by which the impulse to save lives overwhelmed any competing impulse to protect babies from the hazards of clinical innovation. This sort of innovation led to an ethical critique of neonatology on the grounds that the whole endeavor seemed to be experimental in many ways but without the safeguards thought necessary to protect subjects from the risks of such experimentation.

The second era of neonatology was also a time of rapid innovation, but the innovation differed from that in the earlier period. Therapeutic advances continued, but they were less dramatic than those of the first era. The forms of innovation during this era were also more variable. Some were classic randomized trials, others developed and were studied in a less formal manner. In this chapter, we examine the comparative advantages and disadvantages of these two approaches to innovation.

The innovations of this era can be divided into three categories: advances in the treatment of respiratory failure, preventive treatments, and new techniques for monitoring babies.

ADVANCES IN THE TREATMENT OF RESPIRATORY FAILURE

A number of new treatments for respiratory disease in the newborn came into widespread use in the 1980s and 1990s. Most had been in the development pipeline throughout the 1970s. The new treatments included artificial surfactant, extra-corporeal membrane oxygenation (ECMO), high-frequency oscillating ventilation (HFOV), and nitric oxide. The processes by which these various therapies were evaluated and then incorporated into clinical practice were quite different. Surfactant and ECMO, in particular, represent two extreme examples of the processes by which innovation becomes standard treatment. We will examine these two in some detail.

The development of pulmonary surfactant as a clinically useful therapeutic intervention is one of the great success stories of medical science. The chemical itself was discovered in the 1950s. Its role in pulmonary function was elucidated through a series of elegant experiments in the late 1950s and early 1960s. Clinicians immediately began to imagine how it could be used clinically in respiratory distress syndrome of the newborn.

Initial clinical trials of surfactant in the 1960s were miserable failures. Chu and colleagues, working in Singapore, treated fifteen babies with an artificial surfactant.[1] They showed that it did not improve survival, although it did lead to some temporary improvements in lung compliance. The failure of surfactant in the early trial was partly explained by the lack of other supportive treatments. Intubation and mechanical ventilation were not routine in the nursery in Singapore where the trials were conducted. The report by Chu and colleagues was published as a seventy-five-page supplement to the journal *Pediatrics*. It dampened enthusiasm for further clinical trials of surfactant for more than a decade.

The perception that Chu's trial was a failure is as interesting as comparable perceptions of success in clinical trials. Such perceptions are as much a matter of expectation as they are of results. In the case of surfactant, the investigators had unrealistic expectations of what surfactant might do; they designed their studies based on those unrealistic expectations and then had to conclude that the drug had failed. They misunderstood the physiology of neonatal respiratory distress syndrome in that they expected a single dose of exogenous surfactant to cure the disease. Later investigators would come to understand that exogenous surfactant would seldom cure the respiratory distress syndrome. Instead, it only ameliorated the symptoms and made other supportive therapies more effective. Babies treated with surfactant would often still require mechanical ventilation. In the 1960s, however, when the techniques for ventilation and for other supportive care were not well developed, surfactant was a therapy whose time had not yet come.

The perception of failure had spin-off benefits, however. It allowed scientists time to better characterize the physiological properties of surfactant and to conduct a series of animal studies using exogenous surfactant therapy. These studies eventually became the basis for experiments by Fujiwara's group in Japan using exogenous surfactant in babies. In 1980, they published a report of the use of endotracheally administered surfactant to ten premature babies. They wrote, "Oxygenation and alveolar-arterial oxygen gradients improved, the levels of inspired oxygen and peak respirator pressure could be reduced, and many of the radiological abnormalities resolved. Acidosis and systemic hypotension were also reversed. In nine infants a patent ductus arteriosus became evident after recovery from HMD, necessitating further assisted ventilation. Eight infants survived, including five of six with birthweight less than 1500 g; two died of unrelated causes. Postnatal tracheal instillation of artificial surfactant may prove a useful treatment for severe HMD."[2]

These positive results electrified the world of neonatology. As with the earlier trials in Singapore, however, perception was as much a part of the response as reality, as seen by examining the results of a number of clinical trials that were carried out in other centers in the years following Fujiwara's report. Interestingly, the results of those trials are not straightforward or easily interpretable. Kwong's group in Buffalo reported a randomized trial of twenty-seven babies who were born at 24–28 weeks gestation. Half received bovine surfactant, and half received a saline placebo. The treated infants showed immediate improvement in oxygenation and ventilation.[3] Interestingly, these investigators do not report mortality rates or long-term outcomes so, in a sense, their "positive" results are similar to the "negative" results reported earlier by Chu's group in Singapore. Surfactant had not changed, but the world around it had, in the sense that surfactant was now seen as an adjunct to mechanical ventilation, rather than a stand-alone cure.

Raju and colleagues in Illinois reported similar results but also reported improvements in survival among the surfactant treated infants.[4] Shapiro's group in Rochester conducted a similar trial but found no difference in survival between the two groups.[5] These were all small, single-center studies.

In 1989, Horbar and colleagues published the results of a multicenter trial.[6] Their results were much less dramatic than those of the earlier, smaller trials. Although the infants in the surfactant group had a lower incidence of certain pulmonary complications, such as pneumothorax, they did not fare much better in other more important outcomes, "There were no statistically significant differences between the groups in the proportion of infants in each of five ordered clinical-status categories on day 7 ($P = .08$) or day 28 ($P = .75$) after treatment. There were also no significant differences between the groups in the frequency of bronchopulmonary dysplasia, patent ductus arteriosus, necrotizing enterocolitis, or periventricular-intraventricular hemorrhage. In each group, 17 percent of the infants died by day 28." These results, taken at face value, might have been interpreted as "negative," that is, as showing that surfactant did not confer appreciable benefits. That is not how they were generally perceived, however.

A year later, Fujiwara's group published the results of their larger, multicenter trial. Their results were also mixed. Surfactant-treated babies had a lower incidence of some complications but not of others. "Treatment with this surfactant resulted in a significant reduction in the severity of RDS with a concomitant increase in the proportion of neonates with mild disease. The frequency of pulmonary interstitial emphysema and of pneumothorax was significantly lower in treated neonates compared with control neonates. The frequency of intracranial hemorrhage (20%) was significantly lower in the surfactant group compared with the control group (54%, $P = .0008$) and was also reduced for the smallest neonates in the surfactant group (13% vs. 73%, $P = .00008$)." There were no differences between the groups with respect to the frequency of patent ductus arteriosus, pulmonary hemorrhage, necrotizing enterocolitis, sepsis, retinopathy of prematurity, or, most importantly, death.[7] The authors suggest that the improvements that they achieved with a single dose might be magnified if multiple doses were given.

In spite of these somewhat mixed results and in spite of the lingering uncertainty about the appropriate dose, timing, or type of surfactant, the Food and Drug Administration (FDA) approved the use of the first synthetic formulation of surfactant in 1990. The approval took place in record time—just five months from the initial application until the approval was announced—suggesting that the perception of benefit derived from various studies outweighed any evidence suggesting caution. Over the next decade, other forms of surfactant would be approved, further studies would be carried out to compare the safety and efficacy of one formulation with another, and different treatment regimens would be evaluated.

Artificial surfactant was one of the few drugs to ever be specifically developed to treat diseases of the newborn. By contrast, most drugs that are used in the NICU were developed for, tested on, and approved for the treatment of adults or older children. Thus, most were never rigorously tested in neonates. Instead, they were, and are, used in an ad hoc, off-label fashion. Surfactant, by contrast, underwent the rigorous testing for safety and efficacy required by the FDA approval process. Nevertheless, significant controversies persist about the relative risks and benefits of different surfactant formulations, different treatment regimens, and the net effect of surfactant on survival rates or long-term outcomes. In one sense, these controversies do not seem to matter. Overall, birthweight-specific mortality rates steadily dropped throughout the early 1990s, the years when surfactant use increased. This temporal association allowed the conclusion to be drawn that surfactant was one reason for the decline. However, the rate of decline in the 1990s was no different from the rate of decline in the earlier decades, and there were many other innovations during that time period. It is hard to know whether, without surfactant, there would have been similar measurable differences in birthweight-specific survival rates.

Despite these theoretical concerns, it appears that the story of surfactant comes as close as possible to the paradigmatic scientific approach to the development of a new clinical intervention. Basic science work led to animal studies; animal studies led to human studies; human studies were multicenter, placebo-controlled randomized trials; and results were analyzed quickly, published, and became the basis for regulatory approval and incorporation into clinical practice.

The process by which another innovative treatment for respiratory failure was introduced was quite different. Unlike surfactant, ECMO was not a new drug. Instead, it was a technique that used modified machinery from the operating room and recovery room, along with some innovative surgical techniques, to provide long-term cardiopulmonary bypass and oxygenation of the blood outside of the patient's lungs. This was first described by Bartlett and colleagues in a report published in 1976. As with the early trials of mechanical ventilation, they described their initial patients as "moribund." In their first paper, they report that 4/13 such moribund infants survived. Follow-up papers showed improved survival rates. By 1982, they were reporting 56 percent survival rates among infants who were referred by neonatologists because all other therapies had failed.[8]

With surfactant, early clinical success led immediately to randomized clinical trials. These were stimulated, in part, by the recognized need for such trials to win FDA approval for the new drug. Manufacturers of the drug, who stood to profit from it, sponsored many of the surfactant trials. ECMO, by contrast, was not a drug, did not require FDA approval, was not patentable. It was, therefore, unlikely to be profitable for any particular company. There was, then, neither the financial support, legal need, nor regulatory incentive for the sorts of multicenter, randomized trials that were the hallmark of surfactant's development.

Instead, ECMO developed much the way similarly noncommercial innovations like mechanical ventilation or TPN had developed in the 1960s and 1970s. Different centers learned the techniques of ECMO and applied them to different populations of patients on the basis of their own clinical judgments about the risks and benefits of this invasive procedure. Most of the early reports were small, single-center studies. Many showed results that were more dramatic and successful than the early results of surfactant trials.

Some physicians criticized the approach of Bartlett's group because they relied on historical data to determine eligibility. For example, Dworetz and colleagues at Yale analyzed outcomes for babies in their NICU to see whether the criteria Bartlett's group used to determine that an infant was "moribund" and therefore eligible for ECMO would, in fact, accurately predict death in another NICU, where "standard" therapy continued because ECMO was unavailable. They found that, in the early 1980s, 65 percent of such babies survived. By the late 1980s, 88 percent survived. On the basis of this data, they questioned whether Bartlett's description of these babies as "moribund" was accurate. They wrote, "A conservative ventilatory approach to the therapy of persistent pulmonary hypertension may provide a viable, less expensive, and possibly safer alternative to ECMO."[9]

Two small, controlled trials of ECMO were eventually carried out in the United States.[10] Both used unusual and unorthodox study designs, so neither study convinced skeptics that ECMO was superior to conventional mechanical ventilation. Then, a large, multicenter randomized trial was conducted in Britain that showed the decisive advantage of ECMO over mechanical ventilation, "63 (68%) of the 93 infants randomized to extracorporeal membrane oxygenation survived to 1 year compared with 38 (41%) of the 92 infants who received conventional management. Of those that survived, one infant in each arm was lost to follow up and the proportion with disability at 1 year was similar in the two arms of the trial. One child in each arm had severe disability."[11] While this study seemed to end skepticism about the potential value of ECMO, it did not resolve controversies over the precise indications for treatment. Instead, different centers continued to use different eligibility criteria and to report their results to the ECMO registry that Bartlett had established.

The use of ECMO grew in the late 1980s and then dropped off in the 1990s. In 1988, the ECMO registry at the University of Michigan reported that fifty-two centers were using ECMO. By 1993, there were one hundred such centers. Then growth stopped, and by 1997, the number of centers had fallen to ninety-six. In 1991, ECMO centers treated an average of eighteen patients per year. By 1997, the number was down to nine. These shifts are partially explained by changes in alternative therapies. Many more babies were treated with high-frequency oscillatory ventilation and nitric oxide, therapies that may have averted the need for ECMO. Clinicians were incorporating these unstudied, nonvalidated, but apparently useful, therapies into their clinical algorithms. These trends suggest that, while ECMO was never studied as rigorously or as formally as surfactant, it was also not used in a random or unreflective way; practitioners seemed to adjust their practice patterns to the changing alternatives that were available and to continue to try to use ECMO as a therapy of last resort.

In a sense, the problem faced by physicians who cared for infants with respiratory failure in the 1980s were similar to those faced by Delivoria-Papadopolous and her group in Toronto in the 1960s. In both cases, doctors had to decide when conventional therapy (whatever that was) had failed (whatever that meant) so that the use of innovative therapy (however that was defined) would be considered both clinically and ethically appropriate.

Interestingly, the two approaches to evaluation exemplified by the surfactant and the ECMO stories raise more issues in theory than they do in practice. In theory, we should know much more about surfactant than we do about ECMO because it was studied in a more traditionally rigorous way. In practice, however, there seem to be lingering uncertainties about the best way to use both therapies. In a recent review of surfactant usage, Horbar and colleagues note that actual practices are inconsistent with the practices that are recommended by experts on the basis of their analysis of multiple randomized trials. They write,

> Prophylactic surfactant therapy was not widely practiced in 2000 by either of the 2 measures available to us: administration of the first dose of surfactant within 15 minutes of birth and administration of surfactant in the delivery room. Fewer than 30% of infants received the first dose of surfactant within 15 minutes of birth. At many units, no infants were treated within this time frame, and no infants received treatment in the delivery room. Furthermore, the first dose of surfactant is often delayed beyond 2 hours after birth. At >25% of neonatal units in our study, >30% of the infants who were treated with surfactant received the first dose >2 hours after birth. Thus, current surfactant treatment practices at many units are inconsistent with the evidence favoring prophylactic and early surfactant treatment.[12]

At the same time, there seems to be widespread agreement among experts in different countries about the clinical indications for using ECMO in neonates. As with surfactant, this broad agreement is not total. There is ongoing uncertainty about details, even as there is consensus about the big picture. Writing about ECMO for the Cochrane Database, Elbourne and colleagues conclude, "A policy of using

ECMO in mature infants with severe but potentially reversible respiratory failure would result in significantly improved survival without increased risk of severe disability amongst survivors. For babies with diaphragmatic hernia ECMO offers short term benefits but the overall effect of employing ECMO in this group is not clear. Further studies are needed to refine ECMO techniques; to consider the optimal timing for introducing ECMO; to identify which infants are most likely to benefit; and to address the longer term implications of neonatal ECMO during later childhood and adult life."[13]

It seems as if the two radically different approaches to the evaluation of these two therapies have led to a relatively comparable degree of clinical consensus. For both therapies, most clinicians in most countries would agree about the current clinical indications. For both therapies, there are outstanding questions about some particular, unusual cases. And, for both therapies, further research continues.

What do these parallel stories tell us about the innovation in clinical neonatology? First, the two treatments—surfactant and ECMO—are very different in nature and they are used for very different populations of babies. As a result, drawing comparisons between the two is not straightforward. Surfactant is a preventive treatment given to all babies below a certain gestational age or birthweight. It is relatively noninvasive and nonburdensome. It does not require ongoing monitoring, a trained team of professionals on call, or dedicated physical space and machinery in the ICU. ECMO is not a discrete intervention so much as it is a commitment of a large group of people to provide an ongoing, high-risk, high-tech life-support device that requires an extraordinary commitment of time, energy, equipment, and money. Surfactant is provided to many babies; ECMO to just a few. At the time each was developed, it was unclear whether the benefits would outweigh the risks. Both required significant changes in the organization and structure of delivery rooms and NICUs to make sure that babies were treated in a timely manner. So comparisons between the two, while not straightforward, are not irrelevant.

Three conclusions can be drawn from such comparisons. First, randomized controlled trials (RCTs) may be better suited for some sorts of clinical interventions than for others. They are most useful when a drug is given at one point, and the effect of the drug cannot be measured until a later time. In such situations, the clinical intuitions of the professionals who provide the treatment about whether it is effective are virtually useless. There is no way that they can judge, at the time of treatment, whether the treatment is having the desired effect. Furthermore, many of the immediately observable effects may be bad—the treatment often makes people sicker before it makes them better. In such situations, randomization, blinding, and concurrent controls are essential to determine the positive and negative outcomes of treatment. Cancer chemotherapy is the best example of such an intervention.

In the intensive care unit, by contrast, many interventions have an immediately observable effect on an immediately observable life-threatening condition. Intubation and mechanical ventilation of a gasping, blue baby can lead to immediate resolution of the life-threatening respiratory distress. In such situations, blinding and randomization are much more difficult to achieve or to justify. The moral and emotional demands of the situation may preclude the state of equanimity and equipoise that are required to conduct an RCT.

Second, randomized trials are not the only way to gain information about the efficacy of treatment. While the RCTs conducted on surfactant undoubtedly gave us important information, they also sometimes gave us conflicting information. They resolved some debates but created others. The nonrandomized clinical trials conducted on ECMO did much the same thing-they gave valuable information that could be scrutinized by practitioners and accepted or rejected based on their own critical reading of the literature. This process of evaluation is similar to the process by which many other innovations in neonatology and in other areas of medicine has taken place.

The incremental process of innovation, observation, evaluation, and critical appraisal of innovation is the hallmark of most medical progress. In many cases, this process yields an understanding of the situations in which an RCT is needed. After all, investigators should only participate in an RCT if they are genuinely uncertain about the relative risks and benefits of two treatments. But if one of the treatments is the "standard" treatment and the other is the "innovative," or "experimental," treatment, then investigators already know, or should know, a lot about the risks and benefits of the "standard" treatment. Thus, they must also know a fair amount about the risks and benefits of the innovative treatment to judge it roughly equivalent. However this prior knowledge is obtained, it must allow the possibility that the knowledge will convincingly show that the innovative treatment is likely to be better. Very few neonatologists remained genuinely uncertain about whether intubation and mechanical ventilation were equivalent to supplemental oxygen alone for babies with RDS, even before any RCTs were conducted on this intervention. Thus, randomized trials of mechanical ventilation were not generally a part of the process of innovation and should not have been.

Third, the privileging of randomized controlled trials and the consequent disparaging of information gained by other means may lead to worse, rather than better, evaluation of innovation. That is because the focus on RCTs can discourage thoughtful clinicians from evaluating their own observations and experiences. After all, if the only way to know that something works is by conducting an RCT, then the observations of an individual about the relative risks or benefits of an intervention are useless. However, without such critical thinking by individuals outside of the confines of a clinical trial, the disjunction between what we call "standard practice" and what we call "clinical research" becomes even wider.

This ever-widening gap is reinforced by the regulatory guidelines distinguishing research from practice and the effects that these regulations have on what gets published. To publish, a clinician must first have conceptualized the work as research, sought approval from an IRB, obtained consent from parents or patients, collected the data in a prospective manner, analyzed it in using rigorous statistical techniques, and written it up in ways that conform to these conventional expectations. We saw, in the early papers on neonatal intervention, how these formal stylistic requirements probably led to distortions of actual experiences. By this approach, there is little room for the serendipity, or thoughtful reflection on the lessons that can be learned from careful observation of experience, or the appropriate use of retrospective evaluations of experience that have always been and will likely always be the mechanisms by which new ideas are generated.

Thus, by concretizing the criteria for quality, we may improve the quality of some sorts of clinical research, but we diminish the value and the yield of other sorts of useful appraisal. To put it another way, if every innovation in medicine was subjected to a carefully designed prospective randomized, controlled trial before it was incorporated into clinical practice, we would likely be more sure than we are now about the value of innovations, but we would have far fewer innovations and they would take place far more slowly. The trade-offs between that approach and the current approach are not clear-cut. Both have risks and both have benefits. A more nuanced understanding of the relative merits of each approach might lead to a more balanced approach to the regulation and evaluation of innovation.

PREVENTIVE TREATMENTS

Progress in preventive treatments was another focus of the 1980s . Two preventive treatments, in particular, were developed, evaluated, and clinically tested in the 1980s. One was the use of steroid therapy given to pregnant women in premature labor to hasten the process of lung maturation in the premature baby. The other was the screening of pregnant women for group B streptococcal (GBS) colonization. If transmitted to the newborn, GBS could cause life-threatening infections. Treating the pregnant women with antibiotics was shown to reduce the likelihood of life-threatening GBS infection in their babies.

The stories of these two interventions are interesting because they illustrate a curious and often overlooked aspect of innovation in neonatology and other areas of medicine. In contrast to the innovative exuberance in the absence of good evidence that characterized ECMO, or the carefully conducted RCTs that characterized surfactant, these innovations were carefully studied and shown to be effective but were nevertheless not adopted by most obstetricians or pediatricians. They illustrate another feature of medical innovation. Not only does much innovation take place without careful study; much careful study does not lead to appropriate change in clinical practice.

The steroid story began in 1972 when Liggins and Howie[14] demonstrated a reduction in the incidence of respiratory distress syndrome and in mortality among neonates whose mothers were given corticosteroids during the last days of their pregnancies. They advocated the widespread use of "antenatal corticosteroids" to prevent the complications of respiratory distress syndrome. After this classic study, more than a dozen similar studies showed dramatic improvements in outcomes.[15] By 1990, Crowley and colleagues collected and reported results of twelve well-conducted randomized trials in nearly 3000 patients showing a 50 percent reduction in the incidence of respiratory distress syndrome and a 40 percent reduction in neonatal mortality. Furthermore, they showed that these reductions in mortality were accompanied by a decrease in morbidity. In particular, they showed that the occurrence of intraventricular hemorrhage, one of the most devastating complications of prematurity, was lower in the newborns whose mothers had been given corticosteroids than in those whose mothers were not treated.[16]

Despite this growing body of evidence from high-quality studies published in peer-reviewed journals, most doctors did not use antenatal corticosteroids. In 1985, only 8 percent of women in preterm labor received such treatment.[17] It was not until 1994, when a National Institutes of Health consensus conference recommended the routine use of antenatal steroids,[18] that practice began to change. Following that conference, change came rapidly. By 1995, 55 percent of women in preterm labor were given steroids. By 2000, the number had risen to 75 percent.[19]

Thus, the 1980s were a decade in which antenatal corticosteroids were shown to be effective but during which it was difficult to convince practitioners to incorporate them into routine clinical practice. The reasons for this professional reticence are somewhat mysterious, especially when compared with the enthusiasm with which practitioners adopted mechanical ventilation and surfactant. Physicians should be more responsive to the evidence derived from well-conducted randomized trials than they are to anecdotal reports. In actuality, however, as the antenatal steroid story suggests, many randomized trials fail to change practice, while many reports of innovative treatment that were not so rigorously studied led to widespread changes in treatment. For example, obstetricians were much more likely to incorporate intrauterine fetal monitoring or pharmacologic attempts to stop labor into their practices in the 1980s, in spite of the lack of good evidence for the efficacy of these interventions,[20] than they were to incorporate the use of antenatal steroids, despite the excellent evidence for the efficacy of this treatment. So it was not simply that doctors were appropriately cautious and unwilling to adopt new practices until multiple careful studies had been done and assessed by experts in the field.

Such sociological observations about the way innovation is carried out and taken up by the medical profession suggest that multiple factors influence physician practice and that they do so in complex and poorly understood ways. Clearly, any robust understanding of medical progress must examine every step of the process, including the production of knowledge through careful scientific study; its dissemination through scientific meetings, published articles, and consensus conferences; and its ultimate uptake by ordinary practitioners in their day-to-day practice.

Many efforts to reform the procedures of medical progress focus on the protection of research subjects. The implication of this focus is that clinical trials in which knowledge is produced constitute the riskiest stage of innovation. The story of antenatal steroid nonuse suggests a flip side of that risk—that patients can also be put at risk of harm by physicians' failures to incorporate new knowledge and information into their clinical practice. Given the dramatic reductions in morbidity and mortality brought about by antenatal steroid use, the failure to adopt this therapy in a timely way led to thousands of potentially preventable deaths and perhaps many more thousands of babies with preventable impairments.

The story of the development of protocols to prevent neonatal infections with maternal GBS has some similarities to the story of antenatal steroids. In pregnant women, GBS often causes asymptomatic urinary tract infections, or "bacteriuria." It can also cause urinary tract infection or infections of the uterus or amniotic fluid. After labor and delivery, it can cause endometritis and wound infections.[21] Mothers who carry the bacteria may be completely asymptomatic but can transmit the infection to their newborn babies. In the newborn, GBS can cause life-threatening pneumonia, sepsis, and meningitis, which result from transmission of GBS during labor or delivery from mother to infant.[22] The Centers for Disease Control and Prevention estimated that GBS caused 7600 cases of sepsis and 310 infant deaths in 1990.[23] These grim facts suggested that any strategy to reduce transmission from mother to infant would be a welcome addition to perinatal care. In 1979, Yow and colleagues showed that giving ampicillin to mothers colonized with GBS dramatically reduced perinatal transmission of GBS.[24]

A number of studies over the next decade showed similar results.[25] The incidence of invasive GBS disease in neonates dramatically decreased at hospitals that implemented screening and treatment protocols.[26] By 1992, the American Academy of Pediatrics interpreted this evidence as definitive. They recommended screening of all pregnant women and treatment of GBS carriers. The American College of Obstetrics and Gynecology interpreted the evidence from the studies differently. They felt that routine screening of all pregnant women would be unnecessary and that, instead, obstetricians should clinically assess their patients and screen only those who had certain risk factors for GBS infection.[27] These two approaches to GBS prevention had very different costs and levels of efficacy. The lack of a consistent professional standard led to widespread confusion and practice variation. Physicians were quite slow to adopt universal screening protocols.[28] It was not until the mid-1990s that obstetricians and pediatricians resolved their differences and jointly recommended a strategy of universal screening, which led to a dramatic decline in neonatal deaths from sepsis. In a national study, death rates were cut nearly in half, from 24.9/100,000 live births from 1985 through 1991 to 15.6 from 1995 through 1998.[29]

The stories of antenatal steroids and GBS screening suggest that the availability of evidence that an intervention is beneficial is often not enough to lead to the intervention's clinical adoption. In both cases, the story may not be over. Recent studies of steroid use in other neonatal clinical situations suggest that it may increase the long-term risk of developmental problems. Widespread use of intrapartum antibiotics to treat GBS colonization may lead to increased antibiotic resistance and more severe infections later in life. In both cases, then, innovation is an ongoing process. Evidence is always suggestive, never complete. The balance between exuberant uptake of an innovation or appropriate caution is always a hard one to find. Such issues become even more confusing when professional societies cannot agree on an interpretation of the data. Many times, in clinical practice, the practitioner must decide among multiple, competing standards of excellence. In a sense, then, much of clinical practice is an ongoing experiment.

OTHER MEDICAL ADVANCES IN THE 1980S

Other than the advances previously described, the 1980s were a decade of refinement in the practical aspects of neonatal intensive care. Neonatal intensive care units grew bigger and busier, nurses gained more experience, and many new monitoring techniques became available that improved the ability of professionals to take care of critically ill newborns. The development of easy-to-use, noninvasive oxygen-monitoring devices in the 1970s,[30] and their widespread clinical use in the 1980s,[31] allowed fine-tuning of ventilator management and the possibility of avoiding some of the consequences of oxygen toxicity. Cranial ultrasonography made it easier to diagnose intraventricular hemorrhages without moving unstable babies from the NICU to the radiology suite. Better intravenous catheters allowed better venous access with fewer complications. Altogether, these changes probably led to as much of an improvement in survival as any discrete therapeutic intervention.

The net result of these medical developments in the 1980s was a steady improvement in survival for babies at every birthweight.[32] Some studies suggested that the survivors had less long-term neurologic problems,[33] but other studies did not show such a trend.[34] These medical developments, though remarkable, were the background against which a national controversy about neonatal care took place. Interestingly, that controversy did not focus on premature babies. It did, however, take for granted the success of neonatal intensive care. Disagreements about the treatment of a particular baby born in Bloomington, Indiana, in 1982, triggered the national controversy.

LEGAL AND POLITICAL ISSUES IN THE 1980S: THE CASE OF BABY DOE

The Baby Doe controversy of the mid-1980s looms over the history of neonatology. The controversy was unprecedented for the way in which a debate about clinical medical ethics, focusing on a single case, engaged the nation. Editorials appeared in major newspapers and magazines. Cases were brought before the U.S. Supreme Court. There were presidential directives and acts of Congress. These led to shifts in the prevailing moral and political landscape that changed the way America thought about the treatment of critically ill babies. To understand the case and all that it came to represent, we will briefly review the medical facts of the case, summarize the legal actions that followed, speculate on the reasons for the political controversy, and attempt to analyze the consequences.

Medical Facts

Baby Doe was born with Down syndrome and a congenital blockage of his esophagus. Down syndrome is associated with mental retardation of varying degrees. A recent review stated, "Individuals with Down's syndrome have a wide range of function in all areas of development. Although in early infancy they function in the range of low typical development, the intelligence quotient decreases in the first decade of life."[35] Life expectancy for individuals with Down syndrome was 49 years in 1997.[36]

Baby Doe's esophageal atresia, with a tracheoesophageal fistula, made it impossible for him to eat. With such a malformation, anything that he swallowed would end up not in his stomach but in his lungs. This is a condition for which surgical repair is routine and routinely successful. Without a surgical repair of this congenital anomaly, he would die of either starvation or pneumonia.

A doctor from the hospital where Baby Doe was born offered these facts about the clinical course in a letter to the *New England Journal of Medicine:*

> The birth weight was 2722g and the length 50.8 cm from crown to heel. The presence of Down's syndrome was readily apparent from the flat nasal bridge, broad epicanthal folds, upward-slanting eyes, and rounded calvarium. A catheter could not be passed into the stomach, suggesting tracheoesophageal fistula, and chest x-ray films revealed a somewhat enlarged heart, which—together with decreased pulses in the extremities—led to a diagnosis of possible aortic coarctation.
>
> After consideration of all the medical information the parents decided not to authorize surgery. The infant was given phenobarbital (5 mg) and morphine (2.5 mg) as needed for pain and restlessness. The parents visited and held the child frequently until his death six days later.[37]

Legal Facts

The facts of the legal case that followed the birth of Baby Doe have been summarized by Meisei as follows:

> In April, 1982 . . . the parents of a newborn infant with Down's syndrome and tracheal-esophageal fistula declined repair of the fistula . . . The parents felt that 'a minimally acceptable quality of life was never present for a child suffering from such a condition,' and further that it was not in the best interests of the infant, their other two children, and the family entity as a whole for the infant to be treated. The hospital in which the baby was born filed an emergency petition seeking to have the parents' refusal of surgery overridden.
>
> The court heard testimony from the mother's obstetrician that he and other members of the obstetrical group believed that the infant should remain at the hospital

where he was born, knowing that surgery was not possible there and that the child would soon die. This recommendation was based on the fact that 'even if surgery were successful, the possibility of a minimally adequate quality of life was non-existent due to the child's severe and irreversible mental retardation.' The infant's pediatrician and a pediatric consultant, although agreeing with the obstetrician's prognosis, recommended in testimony that the infant be immediately transferred to another hospital where corrective surgery could be performed.

In a one sentence conclusion, the trial court determined that the parents, having been fully informed of the available alternative courses of treatment, 'have the right to choose a medically recommended course of treatment for their child in the present circumstances.' However, it also appointed local child welfare authorities as the child's guardian ad litem to determine whether to appeal the case. They decided not to do so. The district attorney petitioned the juvenile court to determine whether the infant was neglected under state law. This petition was denied, and a writ of mandamus in the Indiana Supreme Court was dismissed as moot because of the child's death.[38]

Social and Political Ramifications

That might have been the end of the story, as it had been the end of so many such stories before, had not a constellation of political and social forces conspired to elevate this particular baby into a cultural icon.

The early 1980s were a time when the science of neonatology was mature enough so that the political and economic infrastructure supporting it solidified. Neonatology had become mainstream. Most states had developed regionalized perinatal systems. Neonatology became a bona fide subspecialty of pediatrics, with its own national board, exam, and certification. The medical advances of the 1970s, including mechanical ventilation and parenteral nutrition, were no longer considered innovative or experimental. Birthweight-specific survival rates were steadily improving.

These were also the years when many of the political and social changes of the 1970s, seen as radical and transformative, came to be viewed as more mainstream. By the time Baby Doe was born, it had been nearly ten years since the U.S. Supreme Court decision in *Roe v. Wade* legalized abortion throughout the United States, since the Rehabilitation Act of 1973 enshrined the right of disabled Americans to be treated fairly, and since federal legislation recognized the need for state child protection agencies to insure that children were not abused or neglected.

These were also the early years of the Reagan administration, which had promised to change the direction of national policy. President Reagan had been elected with overwhelming support from the religious right, a group that was eager to overturn *Roe v. Wade* and to protect what they saw as the sanctity of human life, including the lives of the unborn.

Leaders within the Reagan administration were troubled by the story of Baby Doe. The President himself asked aides to find a way to use federal law to prevent such cases from happening again. In an article entitled, "Abortion and the Conscience of the Nation," Reagan wrote of the case:

> What more dramatic confirmation could we have of the real issue than the Baby Doe case in Bloomington, Indiana? The death of that tiny infant tore at the hearts of all Americans because the child was undeniably a live human being—one lying helpless before the eyes of the doctors and the eyes of the nation. The real issue for the courts was not whether Baby Doe was a human being. The real issue was whether to protect the life of a human being who had Down's Syndrome, who would probably be mentally handicapped, but who needed a routine surgical procedure to unblock his esophagus and allow him to eat. A doctor testified to the presiding judge that, even with his physical problem corrected, Baby Doe would have a "non-existent" possibility for "a minimally adequate quality of life"—in other words, that retardation was the equivalent of a crime deserving the death penalty. The judge let Baby Doe starve and die, and the Indiana Supreme Court sanctioned his decision.[39]

Finding a mechanism by which the federal government could intervene was not straightforward. No obvious regulatory apparatus gave the federal government any oversight of medical decision making for babies. The Justice Department eventually proposed a controversial mechanism for intervening. They defined decisions like the one made for Baby Doe as discrimination against children with disabilities, a violation of federal civil rights laws. Any organization that was found to be in violation of civil rights laws could lose all of its federal funding. For hospitals, this potentially meant that they could lose their Medicare, Medicaid, and National Institutes of Health funding. The president described this as follows:

> Federal law does not allow federally-assisted hospitals to decide that Down's syndrome infants are not worth treating, much less to decide to starve them to death. Accordingly, I have directed the Departments of Justice and HHS to apply civil rights regulations to protect handicapped newborns. All hospitals receiving federal funds must post notices which will clearly state that failure to feed handicapped babies is

prohibited by federal law. The basic issue is whether to value and protect the lives of the handicapped, whether to recognize the sanctity of human life. This is the same basic issue that underlies the question of abortion.[40]

The ironies and complexities of this regulatory effort were deep and profound. President Reagan had not been known for vigorous enforcement of civil rights legislation before this. He had, for example, opposed the Voting Rights Act of 1965, a centerpiece of the civil rights movement. He also had argued that segregated private schools should have tax-exempt status, an argument that most civil rights advocates opposed. And just a year before the Baby Doe controversy, the newly elected Reagan administration tried to amend or revoke regulations implementing Section 504 of the Rehabilitation Act of 1973, the very law he was now invoking to justify a dramatic expansion of federal powers. After the Baby Doe controversy had subsided, the Reagan administration would once again try to limit the reach of Section 504 of the Rehabilitation Act by vetoing the Civil Rights Restoration Act of 1987, a law that extended the scope of federal civil rights law, including Section 504 of the Rehabilitation Act of 1973. Congress overrode that veto.

In spite of these apparently contradictory administrative impulses, the Reagan initiative to use the Rehabilitation Act to change the prevailing paradigms of decision making for imperiled newborns led to interesting shifts in political alliances. For pediatricians, the Reagan regulations were a mixed signal. On the one hand, they seemed to represent an unprecedented endorsement of medical intervention for critically ill newborns. Neonatologists had been arguing for years that newborns had a right to medical care equivalent to that of all other citizens. The Baby Doe regulations enshrined that right in federal law. Thus, it would be no small thing to oppose the regulations. Nevertheless, the regulations also represented an unprecedented intrusion of the federal government into the doctor-patient relationship. Many pediatricians opposed the regulations on those grounds, even as they sympathized with the moral impulse behind them. A spokesman for the American Academy of Pediatrics wrote, "I don't really oppose proper intervention for any child, but I do have deep concern about the propriety of the kind of federal involvement that has taken place so far, such as hotlines, the posting of signs in hospitals, and Baby Doe squads that go rushing into hospitals to check on cases. Such methods are an insult to the intelligence of professional people and a serious threat to the privacy and confidentiality of families in agonizing circumstances."[41]

Opponents of big government generally opposed the regulations on the principle that smaller government was always better. Thus, the *Wall Street Journal*'s editorialists excoriated the administration, writing, "It is indeed ironic. We are well into commemorating the year of George Orwell's famous novel 1984 and the most significant new example of the sort of government intrusion Orwell warned against is being pushed by the conservative administration of Ronald Reagan. We have in mind the Reagan-inspired "Baby Doe" regulations."[42] And the British business newsmagazine, *The Economist,* worried about who would pay for the care of these babies, "The problem that nobody has addressed is who is to pay the costs of looking after children who are saved. The medical costs, which are likely to be large, could be met by the federal government. But over the years there will be a heavy price to pay if the child grows up in an institution . . . Perhaps the right-to-life lobbies will chip in."[43]

The mainstream liberal press also opposed the regulations. A *New York Times* editorialist worried that "the medical attention that should be given to a badly damaged baby is not something to be determined by someone untrained to understand the problem, let alone the answer." The *Times,* like the *Wall Street Journal,* recommended that hospital ethics committees should be empowered to oversee such decisions, using the criteria articulated by the president's Commission on Bioethics. By those criteria, "treatment is only discontinued when the indicated handicaps 'are so severe that continued existence would not be a net benefit to the infant.' "[44] Oddly, the *Times* admitted that, by such criteria, Baby Doe himself should have been treated and was not. Nevertheless, they opposed efforts to enforce such standards legally.

Civil libertarian Nat Hentoff highlighted the contradictions of these liberal views. He wrote an essay entitled, "The Awful Privacy of Baby Doe" in which he highlighted the hypocrisy of those who (1) favored standards; (2) noted the evidence that the standards were not being applied; (3) but didn't support efforts to enforce the standards. He noted, "In Baby Doe cases, after the whistle has been blown by a nurse or a right-to-life organization, not once has a ACLU affiliate spoken for the infant's right to due process and equal protection under the law. Indeed, when the ACLU has become involved, it has fought resolutely for the parents' right to privacy. Baby Doe's own awful privacy, as he or she lies dying, is also thereby protected."[45]

One key group of people who became a sort of political and journalistic swing vote were the advocates for people with disabilities. The American Coalition of Citizens with Disabilities, the Association for Retarded Citizens, the Association for the Severely Handicapped, the Disability Rights Education and Defense Fund, and similar groups all supported the guidelines. It was surprising for these groups to find themselves aligned with the Reagan administration and the religious right. It was also surprising for many traditional liberals to find themselves opposing groups advocating for the rights of people with disabilities. Pediatricians too were in the uncomfortable position of opposing groups who claimed to be advocates for the rights of children. In doing so, pediatricians were accused of abrogating those very rights.

From this analysis, it can be seen how two of the key political players in the Baby Doe debate—the right-to-life groups who made up Reagan's base and the advocates for the rights of the disabled whose interests uniquely coincided with government policy on this one issue—were groups whose origins lay in the social change of the late 1960s and early 1970s. The advocates for the rights of the disabled were trying to extend the political victory that they had won with the passage into law of the Rehabilitation Act of 1973. The antiabortion groups were fighting what they saw as a rearguard action against *Roe v. Wade*. And the pediatricians had to decide whether and how to respond with attention to both the dilemmas of neonatology and their standing as child advocates. In this sense, the Baby Doe debate represented a sort of societal deep breath, a time for a reflective pause in the juggernaut of social change and medical progress that had characterized the 1960s and 1970s. It allowed a re-alignment based on a curious alliance between a powerful but enigmatic president and two relatively marginalized interest groups who were knitted together by the issue of medical treatment for newborns with life-threatening illness or syndromes associated with cognitive or physical problems.

THE ULTIMATE LEGAL FATE OF THE BABY DOE REGULATIONS

Ultimately, the U.S. Supreme Court struck down the Baby Doe regulations. The case that the court examined involved a baby born with spina bifida whose parents did not consent to surgical repair of the open spinal cord lesion. In reviewing the relevance of the Rehabilitation Act of 1973 to this case, the court focused on the key passage of that piece of legislation, which reads, "No otherwise qualified handi-capped individual in the United States . . . shall, solely by reason of his handicap, be excluded from participation in, or be denied the benefits of, or be subjected to dis-crimination under any program of activity receiving Federal financial assistance."[46]

The administration tried to argue that the decision by the hospital to accede to the parents' request for nontreatment was an example of a citizen being denied the benefits of a program—hospital care—that received federal assistance. Further-more, they argued that the sole reason why she was being denied treatment was be-cause of her anticipated handicaps.

The U.S. Supreme Court focused on the phrase "otherwise qualified." They ar-gued that, in the absence of parental consent, the infant was not "otherwise qualified." Hospitals, they said, could be judged discriminatory only if they refused to provide treatment for which parents did consent. Otherwise, the hospitals would need to override parental authority illegally to treat the baby. Alternatively, of course, they could have gone to court with an allegation of medical neglect, but the doctors in the original Baby Doe case had done just that and the state courts had not taken protective custody. Supreme Court Justice Stevens wrote that the way states investigate or regulate child abuse and neglect protections was "wholly outside the nondiscrimination mandate of Section 504 (of the Rehabilitation Act of 1973)."[47]

Thus, the original federal regulations that triggered so much controversy were, in the end, completely invalidated by the U.S. Supreme Court. Nevertheless, the impulse behind the regulations—to develop, to articulate, and to enforce consistent national standards for nontreatment decisions—led to a profound shift in the moral landscape of neonatology. The private, internally inconsistent, and philosophically muddled standards of the 1970s were recognized as inadequate. The era of unofficial but tacitly acknowledged decisions that were officially illegal but seldom investigated, censured, or punished, was over. However, it was not clear what should take its place.

Attempts to articulate a new understanding led to new public standards for decision making. One version was written into congressional amendments to the Child Abuse and Treatment Act, the law that provides federal support for state child protection agencies. These amendments specified that, to qualify for federal funding, all state child protection agencies had to include in their own rules and guidelines some new rules applying to cases of medical neglect. These amendments thus had limited actual regulatory or legal force. Nevertheless, the language of the guidelines became symbolically important. These amendments specified three criteria for situations in which it would permissible for doctors and parents to withhold or withdraw life-sustaining therapy:

1. The infant is chronically and irreversibly comatose.
2. The provision of such treatment would merely prolong dying, not be effective in ameliorating or correcting all of the infant's life-threatening conditions, or otherwise be futile in terms of the survival of the infant.
3. The provision of such treatment would be virtually futile in terms of the survival of the infant and the treatment itself under such circumstances would be inhumane.[48]

Because the federal government has no official role in policing child abuse, the reach of the Child Abuse and Treatment Act is quite limited. It is a funding mechanism for providing federal dollars to state child protection agencies. The amendments were only suggested criteria for state child protection agencies to use in developing their own rules and regulations for investigating cases of alleged medical neglect and determining whether neglect had taken place. The only regulatory authority of the amendments is to require state agencies to have something like these three criteria to obtain federal funding. Most states quickly wrote some such language, and all qualified for federal funding. The state laws are rarely invoked in actual child neglect proceedings.

More importantly, however, these amendments to the Child Abuse and Treatment Act took on symbolic value. They had, after all, been worked out as a consensus statement by the federal government, the American Academy of Pediatrics, and various advocacy groups for the rights of the disabled. As such, they were as close as we as a country had ever gotten to a formal, politically inclusive, and explicit set of criteria for deciding when it would be appropriate or inappropriate to withhold life-sustaining treatment from a baby.

THE AFTERLIFE OF THE BABY DOE CONTROVERSY: EXPOSED IGNORANCE

In the remaining years of the 1980s, it became clear that the idealistic and inclusive efforts of many groups to achieve a consensus about the principles that should guide decisions about the limitation of life-sustaining medical treatment in newborns had failed. This became painfully clear in a study done by Koppelman and her colleagues who surveyed neonatologists to determine how these doctors might apply the criteria in the Baby Doe guidelines. They presented the neonatologists with three cases. One described an infant with trisomy 13 and congestive heart failure. Trisomy 13 is a chromosomal anomaly that causes severe mental retardation and in which more than 90 percent of infants die before 1 year of age. Twenty-two percent of neonatologists thought that the criteria above would require them to provide treatment for the heart failure, 61 percent did not, and 19 percent were uncertain. A second case described a 550-gram premature baby born at 25 weeks of gestation who develops a large intracranial hemorrhage. Thirty percent thought the regulations would require continuation of treatment while 52 percent did not. A third case described a baby with congenital hydrocephalus, blindness, and severe cognitive impairment. Forty-seven percent thought the regulations required treatment.[49] The rest either did not or were unsure.

This study showed that, in many of the most difficult cases, thoughtful practitioners would disagree about how to interpret the guidelines and might disagree even more about whether treatment ought to be provided or ought to be considered mandatory. The careful regulatory language in the Child Abuse Act apparently would not eliminate practice variation or successfully impose a consistent and universal standard. Part of the reason for this failure is that the language of the regulations implied a level of medical knowledge about outcomes that was largely absent from the clinical practice of neonatology.

Before the 1980s, doctors claimed expertise about three key domains. First, they claimed that they could accurately predict the outcomes for the babies they were treating. In particular, they claimed expertise in determining when further treatment was futile. Second, they claimed that they understood parents' wishes regarding such treatment. Finally, they claimed the authority to understand and evaluate a baby's anticipated quality of life. Claims of such expertise were the foundation of a paradigm for decision making in which the doctors' opinions were given special weight. Many of the doctors' claims turned out to be just wrong, but they could only be proved wrong by data comparing doctors' beliefs to quantifiable facts. Such studies began to be carried out in the 1980s.

One important series of studies documented that many obstetricians, general pediatricians, and even neonatologists had an unduly pessimistic view of outcomes from extremely premature babies. These studies used both assessments of factual knowledge and vignettes to elicit doctors' knowledge and attitudes. For example, Haywood and colleagues surveyed 224 obstetricians in Alabama. They found that obstetricians "significantly underestimated survival rates from 23 through 34 weeks' gestation ($P < 0.05$) and freedom from serious handicap from 23 through 36 weeks' gestation ($P < 0.05$). They advocated early treatment of preterm labor, but <50 percent would perform Cesarean delivery for fetal distress before 26 weeks' gestation."[50]

These underestimations had important consequences for both clinical care and for counseling. Obstetricians who thought that babies could not survive were less likely to provide optimum obstetrical management, less likely to give antenatal steroids to hasten lung maturation in the fetus, less likely to refer pregnant women at a particular gestational age to a tertiary care center, and less likely to have a neonatologist present at the delivery. They may have given parents inaccurate and misleading information about the anticipated outcome for their baby, leading parents to choose nontreatment instead of neonatal intensive care. Thus, their erroneous prognostications could become self-fulfilling prophecies.

Pediatricians and neonatologists, too, were inaccurately pessimistic about outcomes. Lee and colleagues showed that, "Both pediatricians and nurses tended to overestimate the morbidity, mortality, and costs of care of VLBW infants. There was a direct correlation between a negative attitude toward saving VLBW infants and a negatively false perception of neonatal morbidity, mortality, and costs."[51] Such gaps and lags in knowledge reflected that absence of any large, well-publicized multicenter studies that would allow practitioners timely access to relevant outcome data.

There were many reasons why such studies were not conducted. Throughout the 1970s and in the 1980s, clinicians viewed outcome studies with skepticism because the inevitable time lag between initial treatment of a baby and the measurement of long-term outcome made the studies seem dated or obsolete. Any study with a five-year outcome, for example, would take more than five years to be conducted, completed, and published. The results of such studies would indicate what the outcome would be for babies who had been born six, eight, or ten years before. Practitioners could plausibly claim that improvements in neonatal treatment would lead to better outcomes for current babies than those described in the outcome studies of babies who had been born five or ten years before.

But the problems went deeper than concerns about outdated results. Pediatricians also had unrealistic expectations about their own prognostic abilities. This is best illustrated in the debate about the concept of medical futility. At first, the concept of medical futility seemed like a simple and uncontroversial place to start in defining situations in which withholding or withdrawing treatment would be appropriate. After all, it seemed as though doctors should know whether particular treatments in particular circumstances were efficacious or futile. If futile, they should not be provided. However, attempts to operationalize futility demonstrate how difficult prognostication could be.

One of the lasting legacies of the Baby Doe debate was the key role it played in highlighting the complexities of the concept of "medical futility." Before the use of this concept in the amendments to the Child Abuse and Treatment Act, there had been little recognition of the implications of a decision by doctors that further treatment might be futile. To be sure, there had been discussions of this concept in more ancient texts on medical ethics. Hippocrates, for example, cautioned physicians not to treat patients who were "overmastered by their disease."[52] Many religious traditions acknowledged a shift in moral obligations as death approached. In modern times, the development of palliative care and medical hospices for the dying was, for many, an acknowledgment of the limitations of medicine and recognition of situations in which life-prolonging treatment could be counterproductive. However, it was not until the Baby Doe debate that federal legislation included the concept of futility as a specific criterion that would be necessary before the goals and obligations of physicians and parents should shift.

This triggered a movement to define the circumstances under which further life-prolonging treatment could reliably be deemed futile. The public discussion began with a case report and ethical analysis in the *New England Journal of Medicine* of a case in which a patient who was dying of metastatic cancer requested CPR. Her doctor thought that CPR would be futile. The question was whether patient autonomy, in such a case, should override the physician's opinion that the treatment would be painful, expensive, and unsuccessful.[53] Scores of articles and a number of books followed.[54]

The vigorous debate about the concept of medical futility turned more on definitional issues than on moral ones. That is, there was widespread agreement on the basic moral principle that futile treatments need not be offered. There was widespread disagreement about how to operationalize that principle. To operationalize the principle, it would be necessary to decide exactly what sorts of treatments, for what sorts of patients, under what sorts of circumstances could reliably be deemed futile. In the absence of data, most doctors and hospitals developed policies that were heavy on procedural components and light on substantive components. For example, treatments could be deemed futile when two doctors said they were futile. But reliance on these sorts of procedural definitions was exactly the sort of problem that the attempt to develop objective standards was meant to supersede.

The implications of prognostic uncertainty with regard to survival were significant. Prognostication regarding neurological impairment among survivors was even thornier. Nancy Rhoden, a law professor, summarized the problem well. She wrote, "The difficulty, of course, is in making accurate predictions. Extremely premature infants are very susceptible to intraventricular hemorrhages—bleeding in the brain. Many British doctors said that a few years ago they would have withdrawn treatment from a baby having a Grade IV hemorrhage—the most severe level—because it is highly correlated with death or profound brain damage. But recent data have shown that some infants may be only mildly impaired by even a Grade IV bleed if it is relatively localized within the brain."[55]

Rhoden concluded:

> Sometimes treatment will yield an infant so devastatingly disabled that death would have seemed preferable. Likewise, doctors may withdraw treatment from a baby who possibly could have survived relatively intact. Doctors will agonize over decisions. Parents will agonize as well . . . Doctors and parents may later regret their decision or be tormented by it. This agonizing, however, is only commensurate with the tragic nature of these dilemmas. In fact, those approaches that minimize it may be inappropriate for precisely that reason. When medical uncertainty leads to moral uncertainty, it seems preferable, albeit harder, to confront these dual ambiguities than to bury them under either statistical criteria or unrelenting moral certitude.[56]

Jeff Lyon, a journalist, put the dilemma more graphically, "If it is hard to justify creating blind paraplegics to create a number of healthy survivors, it is equally hard to explain to the ghosts of the potentially healthy that they had to die in order to avoid creating blind paraplegics."[57]

One implication of doctors' inaccurate prognostications was a recognition of the need to include parents in these decisions in a new and different way. In the 1970s, doctors assumed that they understood what was an acceptable and what was an unacceptable quality of life. Following Silverman, Shaw, Duff and Campbell, they also assumed that parents trusted them, shared their values, and did not want aggressive life-sustaining treatment for their babies if the prognosis for neurologic outcome was poor. It turns out they were wrong, both about their understanding and assumptions about what parents wanted. For many pediatricians, this was one of the biggest surprises in the Baby Doe debate. Studies in adults with disabilities,[58] in adolescents who with lifelong disabilities,[59] and in parents of children with disabilities, all show that doctors overestimate the impact of particular disabilities on people's subjective assessments of their own quality of life. Doctors tend to assume that physical and cognitive impairments lead to poor quality of life. Patients and parents report that quality of life is much more related to social support, leisure-time activities, and the perceptions of others than it is to intrinsic factors like physical or cognitive abilities.

These self-assessments of quality of life by people who live with particular disabilities or by parents who care for children with such disabilities are the closest we can get to a gold standard for calibrating quality of life. They cannot be dismissed as ill-informed or swayed by emotion. Parents do not deny the severity of the conditions their children have or the emotional stresses that caring for such children may create. They recognize that their children have special needs and sometimes are severely limited in what they can do. However, they do not associate this with a lower quality of life. As Saigal and colleagues write, "ELBW children were reported to have a greater burden of disability than were control children based on parental descriptions. Nonetheless, parents of ELBW children, on average, rated the health-related quality of life of their children fairly high. Thus, differences in reported functional status are not necessarily associated with lower utility scores."[60] Similarly, Siperstein and colleagues studies doctors' attitudes toward babies with hydrocephalus, and reported,

> Significantly fewer pediatricians would present information to parents in an encouraging light, and significantly fewer would treat their own child, if the case involved severe hydrocephalus in comparison with no hydrocephalus. Pediatricians'

prognostications were the least optimistic for the infant with severe hydrocephalus and most optimistic for the infant without hydrocephalus, and they were considerably less optimistic than seems justified on the basis of follow-up studies... The major import of the findings is that pediatricians' prognoses reflect, in part, a misconception of the impact of hydrocephalus on children born with meningomyelocele and that these prognoses then have and impact on the pediatricians' decisions concerning treatment.[61]

Perhaps because pediatricians and nurses were systematically pessimistic, they did not accurately appreciate how much their attitudes, knowledge, and beliefs differed from those of parents. Generally speaking, parents are more likely to be hopeful about outcomes for tiny babies and to believe that their own baby will beat the odds. Thus, Streiner and colleagues showed that parents were more likely than doctors to favor aggressive treatment of all babies regardless of prognosis tolerant of disabilities than doctors or nurses. They write, "A significant majority of parents believed that attempts should be made to save all infants, irrespective of condition or weight at birth, compared with only 6% of health professionals who endorsed this."[62] This disagreement between doctors and parents is found in studies done in the United States, the United Kingdom, Scandinavian countries, and Australia. It always goes in the same direction.

This robust finding does not, of course, suggest that *all* parents share the same beliefs in these matters or that *all* doctors are pessimistic. It does, however, highlight the likelihood that, if a parent asks a doctor for an opinion about what should be done, the doctor will more often recommend discontinuation of treatment than the parent will be to agree or to accept the recommendation. It may seem unfair to highlight this difference of opinion as an example of pediatricians' ignorance rather than as an example of a legitimate moral disagreement about the appropriateness of treatment in situations where success is unlikely. However, the ignorance here is ignorance of the fact that pediatricians' attitudes are not typical attitudes. With that belief, doctors might assume that parents who want ongoing treatment for a baby with a dismal prognosis are weird, uneducated, in need of counseling, or likely to change their minds. Such studies suggest that none of these are necessarily true.

Quality of life is an inherently problematic criterion because it raises the specter of eugenics or discrimination against people with disabilities. Nevertheless, for most people, a certain minimal level of cognitive or neurological function is essential for them to consider their life to be worth living.[63] This broad consensus emerged strongly during Baby Doe controversy about federal regulation of nontreatment decisions for newborns. There was little disagreement, for example, that for babies who are irreversibly comatose, or babies with chromosomal anomalies that caused severe mental retardation, treatment should not be obligatory. However, the agreement that, in principle, cognitive function is an important consideration, begs the question of what the appropriate threshold for minimally acceptable cognitive function should be. Babies with no cortical function at all, such as babies with anencephaly or babies with prolonged cortical unresponsiveness as a result of anoxic injuries, define one extreme. Babies with syndromes such as Down syndrome that lead to mild mental retardation are at the other end of the spectrum. In between are babies with other chromosomal or genetic anomalies, babies with intraventricular hemorrhages, or babies with neurological damage following treatment for an acute illness.

Analysis of this range of cases has led to careful attempts to define and measure quality of life. The global concept of "quality of life" can be broken down into four ethically relevant subcomponents, each of which must be considered in these cases. These subcomponents include (1) the anticipated cognitive or cerebral function, (2) the anticipated physical disabilities, (3) the pain and suffering that is associated with the disease, and (4) the burdens of the treatments that will be necessary in the future.

The cognitive or cerebral function is a measure of how well a baby will be able to think. In some cases, such as anencephaly, babies have no functioning brain cortex at all. They are completely unaware of their environment and will never be aware. However, in the newborn period, they are able to perform some of the complex motor functions that are controlled by the brainstem, such as sucking and swallowing. Thus, they are not brain dead. In other cases, such as trisomy 13 or 18, babies have extremely limited cortical function. If they survive, they will never be able to talk, to walk or to perform even simple activities of daily living like dressing themselves or feeding themselves. However, they are aware of their environment and respond to pleasurable and painful stimuli. Other cases are associated with milder mental retardation.

The physical disabilities associated with a condition are often, but not always, separable from the cognitive or neurological disabilities. Many babies will have intact cognitive function but will have other physical disabilities. In severe spina bifida, for example, the spinal cord damage that is the essence of the syndrome often makes independent ambulation impossible. People with cerebral palsy have a wide range of physical impairments that are not necessarily associated with cognitive impairments.

A third part of any assessment of quality of life has to do with the pain and suffering associated with the disease. Some diseases lead to unrelenting pain and suffering. For example, severe epidermolysis bullosa is a disease that causes blistering of the skin over the entire body, including the oral cavity and intestinal tract. Swallowing is impossible. Scarring of the skin leads to contractures of all the joints. Even comfort care is difficult because handling these babies causes pain and exacerbates the condition. In such cases, attempts to prolong life inevitably prolong suffering. In other clinical situations, such as chronic lung disease or some degenerative neurological diseases, the pain and suffering of the disease manifests as chronic air hunger due to the inefficiency of the lungs or the muscles that are necessary for breathing. Some diseases cause chronic seizures. Others lead to frequent painful infections.

The final, related component of quality of life has to do not with the pain and suffering of the underlying condition itself but with the pain and other burdens associated with the necessary treatments. Babies with "short gut syndrome," for example, can survive, but only with indwelling venous catheters placed into large veins in the chest or neck. These "central lines" often become infected and must be replaced. When they become infected, patients must be admitted to the hospital for intravenous antibiotics. Intravenous nutrition often causes secondary problems such as liver failure. In extreme cases, patients are frequently hospitalized to deal with the complications of the treatment, and further treatment predictably exacerbates these complications in ways that cannot be prevented. Another example of burdensome treatment is the provision of mechanical ventilation for babies with progressive and degenerative motor neuron disease. Some such babies are unable to eat, breathe, or talk, but their cerebral cortex is intact, so that they can think. Prolonged mechanical ventilation can extend life for such babies, but the burdens of the treatment may be thought to be high enough that a decision not to initiate mechanical ventilation, or to discontinue it once started, is considered.

By breaking down the concept of quality of life into subcomponents, it becomes possible to analyze which elements are driving the decision. For example, a baby with anencephaly and severe cognitive impairment may not be in pain or require painful or burdensome treatment. A baby with short gut syndrome may have normal cognition.

In each of these areas, there are no bright-line distinctions between acceptable and unacceptable quality of life. In each area, most people can imagine cases that they would put on one side of the line or the other. To the extent that people can agree on the appropriate response to a particular kind of case, that case can become a moral paradigm. Thus, if we agree, for example, that quality of life in Down syndrome is acceptable but in anencephaly it is not, then we can try to decide for other cases whether they are more like Down syndrome or more like anencephaly, or whether the burdens of some new treatment are more like those of lifetime mechanical ventilation or more like lifetime dependence on insulin.

The process of reasoning by analogy to paradigm cases allows flexibility and a certain "give" in the regulatory process. We can have a tenuous societal consensus that covers most, but not all, cases. That consensus slowly shifts over time, and reflects the moral principles, the political compromises, and the economic possibilities within a given society.

Recognition of these widespread and persistent areas of professional ignorance leads to two separable implications. One is that doctors came to recognize that they were not in any way a representative group of citizens. This should not be surprising. Doctors are, after all, selected for medical school based on their own superior cognitive abilities. They live and work in a world in which individualism and self-reliance are supreme values. They do not easily ask others for help or admit their own vulnerabilities. Such people would be expected to have different attitudes about physical or emotional functioning than ordinary citizens.

The second, related implication is that doctors must be extraordinarily careful to study and understand objectively the data on outcomes for babies with particular conditions. This data could serve as a check on their own pessimistic attitudes. To the extent that data are available, they can be presented in a value-neutral way so that parents can make an independent assessment of the desirability of treatment in any particular circumstance. To the extent that data are not available, the problems of communication and bias become more complex. It is hard enough to communicate information when the information is available. When it is not and decisions must be made under conditions of real and irreducible uncertainty, the problem shifts from one of achieving a well-defined communication goal to figuring out what the goal ought to be.

The political maneuvering around Baby Doe issues ended with a whimper, rather than a bang. Although there is a law on the books with criteria for decision making, there have been very few legal cases that actually invoke the law. There are two ways to interpret this lack of judicial attention to NICU cases. One is that such cases are still common but that state child protection agencies are not enforcing their own laws either because they are unaware of such cases or because they choose to ignore them. Alternatively, it could be that doctors and hospitals have incorporated the moral standards of the Baby Doe regulations in relatively straightforward cases such as those involving babies with Down Syndrome or myelomeningocele but not in the more difficult cases of, say, premature babies with chronic lung disease and brain damage.

To the extent that the laws provide clear guidance in the former type of case, doctors can use them in discussions with parents. A neonatologist might say, for example, "It is considered child abuse not to operate on your baby's intestinal blockage, even though the baby has Down syndrome." Most parents do not want to be charged with child abuse and to face a legal proceeding that they know they will lose, so they agree to the surgery without the need for going to court. In such cases, the law has an effect even though the effect is not measurable through the frequency of its use.

In the more complex and ambiguous cases, both doctors and child protection agencies seem to have shown caution. It is as if neither side wants to know what a judge might say—neither side cares to reopen the wounds and the controversy of the mid-1980s, and so there is a tacit agreement to allow some discretion, some practice variation, and some moral diversity in areas where there is no broad moral consensus.

AFTER BABY DOE: PRINCIPALISM YIELDS TO EMPIRICISM

One important development that followed from the recognition by doctors of their own limited knowledge was the creation of standardized, multicenter, longitudinal databases. Two such databases were created in the mid-1980s, the Vermont-Oxford Consortium and the National Institute of Child Health and Development Neonatal Research Network. These collaborative organizations were, in some sense, a response to the vast ignorance that existed about outcomes, practice variations, complications, and other concerns related to premature babies and their families.

The NICHD Neonatal Research Network was created in 1986. The network was established to conduct multicenter clinical trials and observational studies in neonatal medicine. According to the network's Web site, it was created "because many of the treatment and management strategies in 1986 had become standards without being properly evaluated."[64] The original neonatal network consisted of seven clinical centers. It has since grown to include sixteen sites.

Among the areas addressed by the Neonatal Research Network are trials of therapies for sepsis, intraventricular hemorrhage, chronic lung disease, and pulmonary hypertension as well as studies of the impact of drug exposure on child and family outcome. The network has a standardized follow-up program of extremely low birth weight (ELBW) infants (i.e., those infants weighing less than 1000 grams at birth. In addition, the network supports a registry of infants less than 1500 grams at birth.

A second multicenter network, the Vermont Oxford Network, was established in 1988 and became fully operational in 1990.[65] At that time, it consisted of fifty-one centers. By 2003, there were over 400 centers in the network, predominantly in the United States but including centers in Canada, Europe, Asia, Africa, and the Middle East.

The Vermont Oxford Network maintains a database including information about the care and outcomes of high-risk newborn infants. The database provides unique, reliable and confidential data to participating units for use in quality management, process improvement, internal audit and peer review.

One of the first things such networks were able to discover was that there was tremendous variation in clinical practices at different sites. Different sites had significantly different rates of initial intubation, mechanical ventilation, treatment of patent ductus arteriousus, and continuation of mechanical ventilation. The authors concluded, "The data demonstrate important intercenter variation of current neonatal outcomes, as well as differences in philosophy of care and definition and prevalence of morbidity."[66]

The databases also allowed retrospective analysis of the relationship between clinical populations at different centers, variations in practice, and differing outcomes at the centers. For the first time, doctors could begin to compare and contrast their own practices not only with anecdotal reports from colleagues about what others might do, or with published series from a single center, but with data collected in a standardized way from dozens of centers throughout the world. The creation of such databases required a political, economic, and moral commitment by leaders of the field to scrutinize themselves and to allow others to scrutinize their work. As such, it took both trust in one another and courage. Such databases ushered in the third era of neonatal ethics.

CHAPTER FIVE

The End of Medical Progress, 1992 to the Present

During the first era of neonatology, the will to innovate led to the discovery of new knowledge and the creation of both new technologies and new administrative structures. These, in turn, led to a second era in which the focus shifted from exuberant innovation to a refinement of both the technologies and the societal mechanisms by which the use of the technologies was governed. Attempts to regulate these new technologies and to refine and improve them led to recognition of our ignorance about many aspects of these technologies and about the best way to use them. This ignorance manifested itself in seemingly irrational, idiosyncratic, or ill-considered decisions by doctors, parents, and policymakers. These bad decisions were based on good motives and strong beliefs about the rights of babies or their parents, the needs of families, the morality of the medical profession, the pathophysiology of disease, or the efficacy of treatment. Both the new science and the new regulation were tenuous, experimental, and evolving. This, in turn, led to recognition of the need to consolidate knowledge about the efficacy and the outcomes associated with these new technologies, which eventually led to the creation of a unique form of clinical data gathering through multicenter databases.

One of the surprising discoveries made through these databases was that, sometime around the mid-1990s, progress in improving birthweight-specific survival rates came to a halt. Evidence for the end of progress comes from a number of independent sources. Horbar et al. reviewed outcomes within the Vermont-Oxford network for the years 1991–1999. They report data on 118,448 babies with birthweight under 1500 grams from 362 different NICUs around the world. The conclusion from their analysis was that "the crude and adjusted rates of mortality, pneumothorax, intraventricular hemorrhage (IVH), and severe IVH declined from 1991 to 1995, whereas from 1995 to 1999, the rates of mortality, IVH, and severe IVH did not change significantly, and pneumothorax increased." They saw this as the end of "a decades-long trend of improving outcomes for these infants."[1] Their mortality data for babies at each birthweight are shown in Figure 1.

A study by Hein and Lofgren analyzing deaths in the state of Iowa in the 1990s suggested the same phenomenon. They reported that the number of deaths that they considered "medically preventable" had declined dramatically between the early 1980s and the mid-1990s. By the mid-1990s, in their opinion, most deaths were "unpreventable."[2]

We reviewed data from our own NICU at the University of Chicago. Overall, 1142 ELBW babies were admitted to our NICU between 1991 and 2002. Birthweight-specific survival rates improved steadily from 1991 until 1997. After that, they remained unchanged.

This leveling off of survival rates was anticipated years ago by astute observers

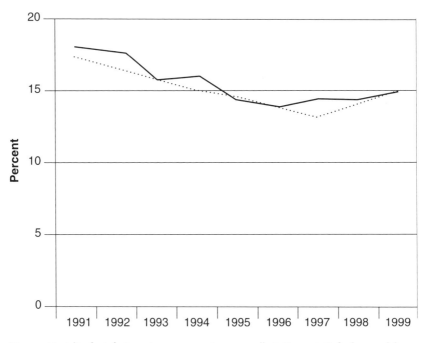

Figure 1 Mortality for infants 501 to 1500 g, 1991 to 1999, at all 362 Vermont-Oxford network hospitals (solid line) and at 39 hospitals participating in all nine years (dashed line). Reproduced with permission from *Pediatrics* 2002;110(1):143–151. Copyright © 2002 by the American Academy of Pediatrics.

of the neonatal scene. Philip studied referrals to a tertiary care NICU between 1982 and 1991 and tried to characterize deaths as "possibly preventable" or "probably unpreventable." He concluded that the number of preventable deaths, given available or foreseeable neonatal technology, was very low. He hypothesized that the only possible way to improve neonatal mortality rates would be to lower the incidence of VLBW births.[3]

Why did progress stop? The clinical innovations that we discussed in the previous chapter—surfactant, antenatal steroids, and treatment of group B streptococcal infections—were the last major innovations in the field. Surfactant was approved by the FDA in 1990 and came into widespread use shortly after that. Antenatal steroid use came to be accepted as standard practice after the consensus conference in 1994.[4] Screening for GBS took off at about the same time. All three of these clinical innovations had been under both laboratory and clinical investigation in the 1970s and 1980s. All were widely implemented in the mid-1990s. Since then, there have been no comparably efficacious interventions in neonatology.

There are two interesting things to note about these innovations. The first is how long it took for them to get from the laboratory bench to the patient. The process of theoretical understanding, animal studies, early clinical trials, consensus conferences, widespread intellectual acceptance, and, finally, widespread changes in routine clinical practice took decades. Given this long lead time for any new innovation to have clinical impact, and the dearth of such innovations on the horizon, it seems unlikely that we will see new and dramatic breakthroughs in neonatology in the near future.

The second issue to note about these developments is that they seem to be the last innovations to truly improve clinical outcomes in neonatology. Of course, there are other innovations that are being tried. Throughout the 1990s, researchers were working on "liquid ventilation," on high-frequency oscillatory ventilation, and on the use of new drugs to improve the treatment of respiratory failure. Some studies have shown some modest benefits from these therapies. Overall, however, birthweight-specific survival rates seem to have leveled off over the past ten years in a way that seems unlikely to change in the foreseeable future. Thus, it appears that the golden era of progress in neonatal intensive care, which lasted from the mid-1960s to the mid-1990s, is over.

The benefits of the innovations made during this period are remarkable. There are roughly 250,000 preterm infants born each year in the United States. Of these, about 75,000 weigh less than 1500 grams at birth. Before 1965, most of these babies died. Today, more than 90 percent of them survive. A conservative estimate, then, is that 20,000 patients per year now survive who previously would have died. Assuming an average life expectancy of about 80 years, that means that neonatal intensive care creates 1.6 million years of life, years that would have been lost without NICUs, every year in the United States today.

The leveling off of progress in neonatology, along with the information from the multicenter databases and from other clinical epidemiological studies, has important implications for our understanding of ethics in the NICU. Because progress has stopped, neonatologists can now, for the first time in decades, offer fairly accurate prognoses for babies born at any given birthweight. Epidemiological research has allowed some refinement of prognostication. At the same time, we have begun to understand the true costs and thus the cost-effectiveness of neonatal intensive care. Legal cases during this period focused, for the first time, on cases involving extremely premature babies, rather than babies with congenital anomalies or genetic syndromes. These cases helped refine societal standards for decision making. Taken together, these developments have led to a widespread consensus about the facts on which moral claims must rest. They have also helped identify areas where further research is necessary.

As in the prior periods, the development of moral norms in this latest period has proceeded in lockstep with the refinement of clinical understanding and the articulation of legal standards. The legal cases in the 1990s were quite different from those in previous periods. They helped define and refine doctors' and parents' understandings of what was or was not permissible.

This decade also saw new attention given to the moral psychology of decision making. There were debates about the proper balance of paternalism and parental autonomy and about how these moral principles should guide discussions about forgoing life-sustaining treatment. In this chapter, we will review each of these areas.

REFINING PROGNOSTIC ACCURACY

Two aspects of prognostication are important in the NICU. Short-term prognostication focuses on the likelihood that a baby will survive the neonatal period or, after that, survive to leave the hospital. Long-term prognostication includes considerations of mortality but focuses more on the chronic impairments that survivors may live with.

Accurate prognostication is the basis for ethical decision making in the NICU. Decisions about whether to continue treatment or to allow a baby to die rely first and foremost on our understanding of the likelihood that the treatment will be successful in staving off death. If we know that treatment will fail, then it is appropriate to discontinue the treatment (or, some might say, inappropriate to have started it in the first place). If, however, we know that treatment will be beneficial, then it is morally obligatory to initiate and continue the treatment. The difficult cases, then, are those that fall between those clear-cut categories—situations in which it is unclear whether the treatment will enable the baby to survive. (Later in this chapter, we will deal with the issue of quality of life for survivors. For now, we focus only on survival.)

From the earliest days of neonatology, population studies allowed us to quantify the overall outcomes for groups of babies. That information helped to define broad classes of babies for whom treatment was either obligatory or futile. The most powerful prognostic measure has always been birthweight. Overall, bigger babies do much better than smaller babies. That is shown, dramatically, in Figure 2. Almost no babies who weigh less than 500 grams at birth will survive, while nearly all babies who weigh more than 875 grams at birth survive. The zone of controversy, then, is between these two weights. They correspond, roughly, to the time between about 23 weeks of gestation and 26 weeks of gestation, or between the fifth and sixth months of pregnancy.

One plausible response to these data would be to suggest that we should treat

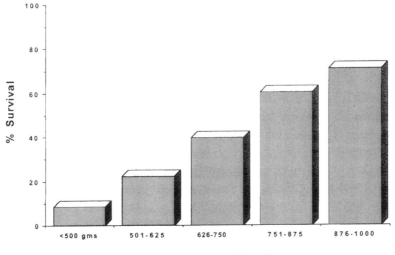

Birthweight (gms)

Figure 2 Survival to hospital discharge as a function of birthweight for 429 extremely low birthweight infants. Number of patients in each birthweight group: 400 to 500 g, n = 32; 501 to 625 g, n = 71; 626 to 750 g, n = 106; 751 to 875 g, n = 107; 876 to 1000 g, n = 100. Reproduced with permission from *Pediatrics* 1996;97(5):636–43. Copyright © 1996 by the American Academy of Pediatrics.

only babies over some specific birthweight. If we treated only babies who weighed more than 875 grams, for example, the success rate of treatment would be quite high. However, as is clear from the graph that, if we were to do that, we would be allowing many babies in the 500–875-gram birthweight range to die who might have survived. If, however, we treat all babies regardless of birthweight, then, as is also clear from the graph, we will provide treatment to many babies whose death is likely.

This sort of information was incorporated in the 1982 President's Commission on Bioethics report on forgoing life-sustaining treatment in neonates, which divided the world of medical treatment into three categories—situations where treatment was clearly beneficial, situations where it was clearly futile, and those in which the outcomes were ambiguous or uncertain. This report suggested that, for babies in the gray zone, parental preferences should determine treatment decisions.

The past twenty years of clinical research in neonatal intensive care has helped us refine our prognostic abilities. One goal of this research has been to develop a method to predict precisely the anticipated outcome for each premature baby, one at a time, case by case. In other words, the goal has been to reduce the domain of the "gray zone" in which all we can say about outcomes is that they are ambiguous or uncertain.

One way to refine our prognostic estimates is to look a little more closely at the clinical course of these babies. What happens if we observe survival rates not just at birth but also at different points in time after birth? It turns out that a baby's initial response to treatment is also an important predictor of survival. The sickest babies, at any birthweight, do not respond to even the most intensive therapy. Other babies, again at any birthweight, respond well to therapy. That initial response turns out to be quite a powerful predictor of ultimate survival.

Figure 3 shows the day of death for all the babies who died in our nursery. In the mid-1990s, more than half of the premature babies who ultimately died would die in the first three days of life, regardless of the treatment that they received.[5] Data from other studies show similar life-course trajectories for premature babies.[6] Because the sickest babies died quickly, the babies who survived for three days were, by definition, much healthier than the others. These data have interesting implications for the timing of decision making about treatment or nontreatment. Specifically, although birthweight is a powerful predictor of survival for all babies who are admitted to the NICU, the predictive power of birthweight diminishes with each passing day. If we look at the association between birthweight and survival not at admission but after three days of age, the graph looks very different. As shown in Figure 4, for babies who are 72 hours of age, birthweight virtually disappears as a

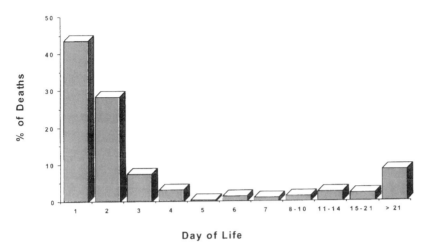

Figure 3 Percentage of deaths as a function of day of life for 227 nonsurviving infants. Reproduced with permission from *Pediatrics* 1996;97(5):636–43. Copyright © 1996 by the American Academy of Pediatrics.

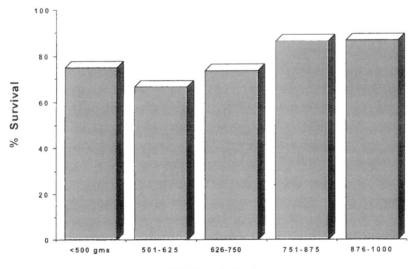

Figure 4 Survival versus birthweight, restricted to extremely low birthweight infants alive on day of life 4. Number of patients in each birthweight group: 400 to 500 g, n = 4; 501 to 625 g, n = 24; 626 to 750 g, n = 57; 751 to 875 g, n = 74; 876 to 1000 g, n = 90. Reproduced with permission from *Pediatrics* 1996;97(5):636–43. Copyright © 1996 by the American Academy of Pediatrics.

relevant predictor of survival. The 600-gram babies who survive for three days do just as well as the 1000-gram babies who survive for three days.

These graphs reflect an important aspect of the clinical reality of neonatal intensive care that has helped shaped the moral responses of NICU professionals. A few decades ago, discussions about the ethics of treatment decisions presumed that the best time to make a decision should be at birth and in the delivery room. The decision about whether to resuscitate in the delivery room was seen as a crucial, either/or, decision that would be irreversible. Once treatment was begun, by this view, it would have to be continued.

The clinical realities that these graphs portray show how that approach is problematic from the standpoint of the baby's interests or from the standpoint of giving accurate information to parents. Among all babies born at less than 750 grams today, half can be saved and half cannot. However, it is almost impossible to tell, at the time of birth, which baby will be in which group. One way to determine more accurately to which group a particular baby belongs is to treat all of the babies. The sickest babies then "declare themselves" by dying in spite of medical treatment. The less sick babies also "declare themselves" by improving over the first few days.

This approach to decision making can be conceptualized as using a "trial of therapy" as a diagnostic tool. It has some interesting implications for our overall understanding of the moral dilemmas of neonatology. First, it makes the process by which prognosis is assessed more complex and time consuming. In the delivery room, the only factor that needs to be considered is birthweight. After a multiple-day trial of therapy, birthweight is no longer the strongest predictor, so a range of other factors must be considered. These factors are less well studied, less well understood, and clearly require an assessment that is more complicated than simply putting the baby on a scale. This process requires all parties to be somewhat flexible and willing to live with uncertainty during the time period during which the assessment takes place. That time period must be flexible because not all babies "declare themselves" at exactly the same time or in exactly the same way. In some cases, babies rapidly deteriorate over 6 or 12 hours. In other cases, it may take days for the prognosis to become clear.

To refine prognostication, researchers have developed multifactorial measures of illness severity. One of the most widely used is the score for neonatal acute physiology, or the SNAP score.[7] This score incorporates a number of physiological and biochemical markers of illness severity to try to categorize babies into prognostic groups. In many ways, the SNAP score has been quite useful. Figure 5 shows the differences in SNAP scores for babies who ultimately survive and babies who ultimately die. At every day of life, the mean SNAP scores are significantly different for

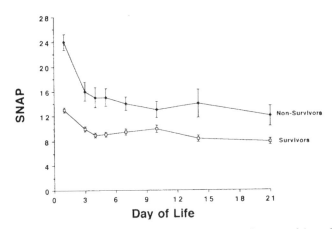

Figure 5 Average score for neonatal acute physiology (SNAP) as a function of days of life
(DOL) for populations of survivors and nonsurvivors during the first 21 days of life. On DOL 1,
SNAP for nonsurvivors (24 ± 8.7 [SD]) was significantly higher than SNAP for survivors (13 ±
6.1; P < .001). This difference diminished steadily over time, as SNAP improved for both groups.
Reproduced with permission from *Pediatrics* 2002;109(5):878–86. Copyright © 2002 by the American
Academy of Pediatrics.

the babies who would go on to die compared with those who would go on to survive. Clearly, babies who die early are sicker than babies who ultimately survive in
ways that this composite measure can quantify.

Although this recognition is helpful, the graph also illustrates one of the problems with using the SNAP score in the clinical context. The scores are most diver-
gent on the first day of life. That is precisely the time when such scores are least
relevant clinically because, as shown above, birthweight by itself is also a powerful prognostic predictor on the first day of life. Later in life, when the predictive
value of birthweight decreases, and the SNAP score could potentially be a more
clinically useful predictor, the differences between the SNAP scores of the two
groups narrow.[8]

Another way to think about the weaknesses of the SNAP score (or other such
objective measures of illness severity) is to look not at the differences between the
mean SNAP scores but at the overlap in scores between babies who would ultimately survive and babies who would ultimately die. This is shown in Figure 6.

Clearly, some thresholds may be useful to predict whether an individual baby
will live or die. For example, on day 3 of life, a SNAP score above thirty seems to be
a reliable and unambiguous predictor of death. However, only two babies fell into
this category. By contrast, babies with a SNAP score between twenty and twenty-
five would be more likely to survive than to die, even though a larger fraction of

babies who ultimately died had a score in this range than of babies who ultimately survived. This is shown, statistically, in Figure 7. This graph shows the positive predictive value, or PPV, of a high SNAP score on each day of life. Colloquially, this is a way of showing whether a SNAP score that is predictive of death is likely to be correct or incorrect. On each day, a high SNAP score is less than 50 percent accu-

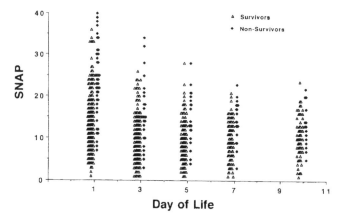

Figure 6 Scattergraph of every SNAP value obtained during the first 10 DOLs for 285 ventilated infants. One hundred twenty-five SNAP determinations for the 45 nonsurvivors and 696 SNAP values for 240 surviving infants are presented. On each day, at virtually all ranges of SNAP scores, at least as many infants will ultimately survive as will die. Reproduced with permission from *Pediatrics* 2002;109(5):878–86. Copyright © 2002 by the American Academy of Pediatrics.

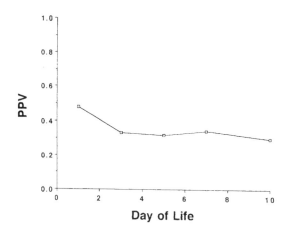

Figure 7 Positive predictive value (PPV) for death of the median SNAP score as a function of DOL. PPV was <0.5 on all days. Reproduced with permission from *Pediatrics* 2002;109(5):878–86. Copyright © 2002 by the American Academy of Pediatrics.

rate as a predictor of death. In short, the SNAP score is more useful as an epidemiological measure of outcomes for large groups of babies than it is as a clinical guide to treatment decisions for an individual baby.

These limitations of quantitative illness severity scores suggest that another approach might be more useful. We recently studied the clinical intuitions of doctors and nurses caring for babies in the NICU to determine whether their gestalt impression of prognosis was accurate.[9] To quantify the accuracy of clinical intuitions, we asked doctors and nurses in our NICU to predict whether babies would live or die. We restricted our study to the sickest babies—those with birthweight of <1000 grams and those who were on mechanical ventilation. For each ventilated infant, then, on each day, we asked doctors and nurses caring for them one simple question: "Do you think this baby will die in the NICU or survive to be discharged?"

Over the course of 18 months, 333 infants were eligible. For 231 of these babies, every doctor on every day that they were in the NICU predicted that they would survive, and they did. These babies exemplify the single most remarkable phenomenon of epidemiology in the NICU. More than two-thirds of all NICU babies who are born at less than 1000 grams and who are sick enough to require mechanical ventilation now survive to be discharged. More important, everybody working with them predicts that they will survive. The highly sophisticated technology of the NICU and the highly experienced staff have taken much of the guesswork out of a situation that was, in the past, mysterious, unpredictable, and usually tragic.

Unfortunately, there's a catch. Although the glass is more than half full, it is not completely full. For the other 102 NICU babies, the clinicians were neither so uniformly optimistic nor so uniformly accurate. These babies were so sick that on at least one day one of the doctors or nurses thought that they would die. What happens to them?

They can be sorted into two groups. One group, about half of the nonsurvivors, were thought by all caregivers to be doomed on every NICU day, and the caregivers were right. The babies died quickly. These were the clinical situations that fell, roughly speaking, into the category of medical futility. There were also babies about whom every caregiver predicted death on at least one day but who did not die, suggesting that the category of medical futility is somewhat porous.

The second group, however, was the most problematic group. It consisted of babies who had at least one NICU day characterized by at least one caregiver predicting that the baby would die but with disagreement among the caregivers. These disparate clinical intuitions were followed by disparate clinical courses. Some of these babies lived; some died. Depressingly, more stringent criteria for prediction of nonsurvival improved predictive power only slightly. Of the babies who had at least one day characterized by two or more respondents predicting death, one-third survived. Of the babies who were so sick that on at least one day every single doctor and nurse predicted that the infant would die, almost one-quarter of these babies still lived to be discharged.

Neither objective, quantifiable measures of illness severity nor intuitive, qualitative assessments by experienced clinicians can eliminate the gray zone of clinical uncertainty. Both prognostic approaches appear best at anticipating impending death only when accuracy does not matter much—for doomed infants with the worst physiology, who will die soon anyway.

What, then, should clinicians tell parents in those situations in which the experts disagree, the prognosis is uncertain, and death seems likely but not inevitable? One response is to try to refine prognostic accuracy not so much by further fine-tuning our predictive accuracy with regard to survival but instead to also consider longer-term outcomes and quality of life for survivors.

PREDICTING LONG-TERM OUTCOMES

Predicting long-term outcomes has all the statistical problems associated with predicting short-term outcomes. In addition, it is fraught with the nonnumeric difficulties of deciding which outcomes are so unacceptable that they might justify a decision to withhold or withdraw treatment. The most troubling long-term outcomes for premature babies involve cognitive or neurological deficits. Premature babies as a group clearly have worse neurological outcomes than full-term babies, and the more premature a baby is, the worse his or her prognosis will be. Numerous studies have shown a higher incidence of cerebral palsy, seizures, and educational problems among premature babies than among their full-term peers. The prognostic problem for clinicians is that, even among the tiniest babies, many survivors have no long-term neurological problems, and there are few good predictors of which babies will or will not have such problems.

Woods and colleagues reported overall outcomes for a group of babies born between 22 and 25 weeks gestation. Their results are displayed in Figure 8. They showed that about half of the surviving babies had no disability whatsoever.[10] Such outcome statistics, however, are like the statistics showing survival rates for tiny babies. That is, they are more relevant for evaluating population outcomes than they are for guiding decisions for a particular baby. For clinicians and parents who must decide whether to continue treatment for a particular baby, the relevant question is

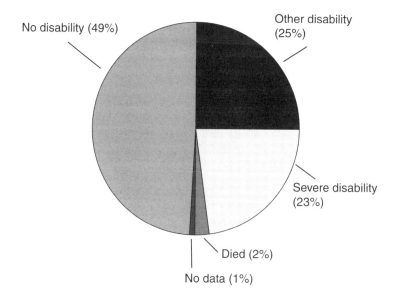

Figure 8 Outcomes for babies born between 22 and 25 weeks gestation in England and Ireland, 1995. *Source*: Wood NS, Marlow N, Costeloe K, Gibson AT, and Wilkinson AR. Neurologic and developmental disability after extremely preterm birth. EPICure Study Group. *N Engl J Med* 2000;343:378–84. Copyright © 2000 Massachusetts Medical Society. All rights reserved.

not, "Of 100 babies like this, how many will have severe disabilities?" Instead, the relevant question is, "Will this baby have a severe disability?"

D'Angio and colleagues tried to refine the prognostic process by retrospectively analyzing which clinical findings are associated with poor cognitive and educational outcomes for babies born at less then 29 weeks gestation. To do this, they followed babies for fifteen years, carefully quantified outcomes, and then analyzed perinatal records.[11] Overall, there were 213 babies born in their NICU during the study period of 1985–87. Of these, 132 (62%) survived to school age, and they were able to evaluate 126 (95%) of these survivors in their early teenage years. At this follow-up visit, 19 children (15%) had cerebral palsy, 24 (19%) were mentally retarded with a cognitive index <70, and 36 (29%) were in special education of some sort. Fifty-one children (41%) had no physical or educational impairment.

They found three predictors of bad long-term neurologic outcomes—neonatal intraventricular hemorrhage, severe lung disease, and low socioeconomic status. Interestingly, these predictors seem interrelated, but they function independently. That is, babies with low socioeconomic status did worse whether they had intra-ventricular hemorrhage or lung disease. At the very least, this suggests a complex interplay between physiological and social factors as determinants of long-term outcome. Such a study, with its fifteen-year follow-up, also highlights the problems with long-term follow-up studies that we mentioned above. These babies were in NICUs in the mid-1980s, before surfactant or antenatal steroids were widely used. The prognosis for such babies may be quite different today, given all the advances of the early 1990s, but we will not be able to know that for another few years.

To get around these limitations, many investigators use shorter time frames for their follow-up studies. Vohr and colleagues found similar results in a multicenter study that followed babies born in the mid-1990s until they were 18 months old.[12] They focused on babies who weighed <1000 grams at birth. At the twelve participating study centers, there were 2498 such babies born during the two-year enrollment period. Of these, 1527 (63%) survived, and they were able to evaluate 1151 (75%) of these babies. Overall, 75 percent of these NICU survivors had a normal neurological exam at 18 months. This included 57 percent of the lowest birthweight survivors, those infants who weighed <500 grams at birth, and 79 percent of those infants who weighed >800 grams at birth. Some of the particular outcomes that they looked at are shown in Table 1.

Shankaran and colleagues analyzed outcomes for babies who shared three markers for high risk of long-term problems: birthweight less than 750 grams, gestational age less than 25 weeks, and 1-minute Apgar scores less than 3. Their study population consisted of 1016 infants. Two hundred forty-six (24%) of these infants survived. Of the survivors, 30 percent had cerebral palsy, 5 percent had hearing impairment, and 2 percent were blind. Nearly half of survivors had significant developmental delay.

We include detailed results of these studies to highlight that neither birthweight nor gestational age was, by itself, associated with poor neurological outcomes for these premature babies. Some of the smallest babies had no clinical complications.

TABLE I

Outcomes for Babies in Different Birthweight Categories, Assessed at 18 Months

Functional Status	Weight Category						
	4–500 g	5–600 g	6–700 g	7–800 g	8–900 g	9–1000 g	Total
n	14	94	205	227	276	295	1111
Sits well alone	64%	87%	83%	86%	85%	88%	86%
Walks	79	79	81	82	83	85	83
Walks fluently	57	64	64	66	72	78	70
Normal arm function	64	89	85	85	86	89	86
Independently feeds self	67	74	74	84	81	85	80

Source: Reproduced with permission from *Pediatrics* 2000;105:1216–26, Table 3. Copyright © 2000 by the American Academy of Pediatrics.

Some of the larger babies had many complications. This again suggests that, in the clinical setting, any simple criterion for treatment or nontreatment based on birth-weight or gestational age alone is likely to be relatively inaccurate and thus ethically problematic in tailoring treatment decisions.

In a follow-up to our study of the accuracy of clinical intuitions to predict survival, we examined whether clinical intuitions might be of more value in this prognostication arena than they were in predicting survival or death.

We now have one-year follow-up data on 187 of the 333 ventilated infants who were in our prediction study.

Of the 83 babies predicted to die, 60 did die. Of the remaining 23 babies who were predicted to die, 16 had definite neurological problems with significant developmental delay, 2 had suspicious neurological examinations, and 5 appeared neurologically intact. Of the 104 babies who nobody thought would die, 24 died before a year of age, 47 (45%) were alive and neurologically intact, and 33 (32%) survived with neurologically deficits.

What can we extrapolate from these observations about extremely low-birth-weight babies? A thought experiment might help. Imagine a cohort of 100 infants who are so sick in the NICU that at least one clinician thinks they will die before discharge. That prediction is likely to be accurate only about 60 percent of the time. This seems woefully inaccurate as a basis for making a decision to withdraw life-sustaining treatment. We now believe, however, that of the 40 surviving infants, only 10 percent will be neurologically intact at a year. This allows a different sort of confidence in counseling parents. They can be told that their baby is more likely to die than to survive, and that if the baby survives, he are she is highly likely to have significant neurological impairment. This seems like a fairly accurate way of defining a "gray zone" in which outcomes are ambiguous or uncertain and in which, therefore, parental preferences ought to guide treatment decisions.

Note, however, that the clinical intuitions require that the baby spend some time in the NICU. As noted above, a trial of therapy gives valuable information in addition to the rudimentary measures of well-being, such as birthweight, estimated gestational age and Apgar scores, that are available in the delivery room. These findings have implications for the process of decision making and would play an important role in a number of legal cases in the 1990s.

LEGAL CASES IN THE 1990S: WHO SHOULD DECIDE?

The slowing of neonatal progress in the 1990s was accompanied by an interesting and related shift in the societal oversight of neonatal decision making. In the

1970s, the oversight of such decision making was mostly private. Doctors and parents made decisions at the bedside. It was unclear whose values or prerogatives drove the decisions, but neither courts, legislatures, nor ethics committees interfered with these decisions. During the 1980s, the federal government tried to exercise some oversight of these decisions through regulatory and legislative activity. This effort had only limited success. During the 1990s, there was very little governmental or legislative activity related to the NICU. Instead, the focus of legal activity shifted from the federal government to the malpractice courts where a number of highly publicized malpractice cases regarding neonatal intensive care became a curious form of policymaking.

The curiousness of such cases was not because of the issues involved. Those issues were generally disagreements between doctors and parents about the proper procedures for and constraints on decision making in the NICU. What made this a curious form of policymaking is the nature of tort litigation. Malpractice cases always turn on the specific details of the case, the strategies of the lawyers, the character of the doctors and parents, and the vagaries of the jury process. As a result, they have a random quality that seems ill suited to the process of public policy formation. Nevertheless, because they also involve large monetary awards, and because they often lead to judicial appeals that then require appellate courts to formulate the legal rationale for decisions, these courtroom dramas often have an effect on medical practice that goes far beyond the letter of the law that they articulate.

The issue in most of the cases of the 1990s was whether and under what circumstances parents have the right to either request that treatment be discontinued or insist that it continue. Such conflicts became legal cases when the disagreements between parents and doctors on these matters could not be resolved using standard techniques of dispute resolution, or when parents decided to initiate litigation long after the events themselves occurred.

One of the first such cases, in 1990, involved a pregnant woman named Carla Miller who sued the Hospital Corporation of America. The case revolved around the events that followed Miller's going into labor at 23 weeks of gestation. Her prenatal ultrasound showed that her fetus weighed 637 grams. She and her husband requested that their baby not be resuscitated or treated. Doctors initially agreed but then, after reviewing the situation with their hospital administration, decided that it would be inappropriate to make a decision before delivery. Instead, they insisted that the neonatologists must evaluate the baby after birth and make a decision based on that evaluation and their judgment about the baby's viability.

Dr. Marc Jacobs, the obstetrician, testified at trial about this decision, "What we finally decided that everyone wanted to do was to not make the call before the time we actually saw the baby. Deliver the baby, because you see there was this [question] is the baby really 23 weeks, or is the baby further along, how big is the baby, what are we dealing with. We decided to let the neonatologist make the call by looking directly at the baby at birth."

Dr. Eduardo Otero, the neonatologist who was in the delivery room, agreed that there was no way to make a good decision before the time of delivery.

The parents continued to insist that treatment not be provided and refused to sign a consent form for treatment. The baby's birth weight was 615 grams. Dr. Otero decided to resuscitate her. He explained why, "Because this baby is alive and this is a baby that has a reasonable chance of living. And again, this is a baby that is not necessarily going to have problems later on. There are babies that survive at this gestational age that—with this birthweight, that later on go on and do well."

The baby's Apgar scores were 3 at 1 minute and 6 at 5 minutes. She was placed on mechanical ventilation and admitted to the NICU. Sometime during the first days of life, she had a brain hemorrhage. The baby ultimately survived with severe neurological impairments.

The parents later sued the hospital, asserting that their daughter was treated without their consent and that the hospital policy of requiring resuscitation without parental consent was illegal. Interestingly, their lawsuit was directed at the hospital, not the doctors.

A Texas jury awarded the parents $60 million. On appeal, the appellate court reversed the decision, stating that parents have the right to refuse treatment on their baby's behalf only if the condition is "terminal," and that, because the baby survived, the condition must not have been terminal. The Texas Supreme Court upheld the appellate court decision, arguing that physicians cannot make assessments of the health or illness of the baby until the baby is born and that, therefore, prenatal decisions may always be reexamined in the delivery room.

The Supreme Court decision held that "the evidence here established that the time for evaluating Sidney was when she was born. The evidence further reflected that Sidney was born alive but in distress. At that time, Dr. Otero had to make a split-second decision on whether to provide life-sustaining treatment. While the Millers were both present in the delivery room, there was simply no time to obtain their consent to treatment or to institute legal proceedings to challenge their withholding of consent, had the Millers done so, without jeopardizing Sidney's life."[13]

This decision presents an interesting interpretation and implementation of the complex epidemiological and prognostic features of prematurity. Most neonatologists would agree with and approve of the court's reasoning. Oddly, however, the decision does not focus on the ambiguous hospital policy that was the actual focus of the suit. The parents and their lawyers tried to focus the case on the issue of whether a hospital could, as a matter of policy, prohibit parents from making a prenatal decision that their newborn should not be resuscitated. The alternative was not a policy that required resuscitation but one that allowed the neonatologist to exercise his own discretionary clinical judgment. The statement from the Texas Supreme Court suggests that they believed Dr. Otero had to have the freedom to make a choice after he'd examined the baby.

It is not clear, because it was not the focus of the case, whether the hospital policy would have allowed him the same option of nontreatment that the Supreme Court insisted he should have. The question that should have been asked of him, and was not, was whether, if he had decided that the newborn baby was not viable or if he thought treatment was futile, he would have been permitted by the hospital administrators to withdraw life support and let the baby die. The court seemed to think that he did have the freedom to make this decision and that he should have had that freedom. The implications of their decision would have been clearer if they had made that conclusion more explicit.

The decision also, of course, does not get into the messy area of trying to decide just what sorts of delivery-room findings ought or ought not lead a pediatrician to decide that resuscitation is morally obligatory. If the reasoning of the Texas Supreme Court is followed to the letter, the only allowable consideration would be the impossibility of survival. There would be no room to consider quality of life, burdens of treatment, costs of treatment, parental preferences, or any other factors. By this reasoning, most modern hospitals would be required to treat all babies above about 23 weeks gestation or 450 grams. Few now do.

Interestingly, in all the testimony in the Miller case, there is no mention about whether there were further discussions between Mr. and Mrs. Miller and the doctors after the initial delivery-room resuscitation. One wonders whether, after the brain hemorrhage, doctors considered withdrawing life support or whether the parents requested it. In an ideal moral world, the prior discussion of parental preferences would have indicated to the doctors that further discussion was important. Unfortunately, in the real world, disagreements early in the course of treatment may lead both doctors and parents to be reticent to bring up such issues later in the course of treatment when the additional data on prognosis might make discussions more fruitful. Furthermore, such discussions sometimes become more emotionally difficult for both doctors and parents even if there have not been prior disagreements between them. The emotional claim that babies make on their caregivers seems to grow over time, regardless of how sick the baby is.

Another important legal case of the 1990s, the Michigan case of Dr. Gregory Messenger and his baby, added a new twist to the canon of case law. In this case, the father did not just request nontreatment of his premature baby. He actually made the decision himself and removed his baby from the mechanical ventilator. He was able to do so, in part, because he was a physician. The case differed from others in that it was not a malpractice case against the doctors but a criminal proceeding against the father who was charged with manslaughter. The facts of the case were summarized in the *Detroit Free Press:*

> In February, 1994, Gregory Messenger, an East Lansing dermatologist, and his wife Traci were expecting their second child. Ms. Messenger went into labor on the morning of February 8, 1994, when the pregnancy was only 25 weeks' gestation. That morning and afternoon her obstetrician administered various drugs to try to slow or stop labor. Ultrasound confirmed a 25-week fetus.
>
> At 6:30 p.m., Dr. Padmani Karna from the NICU staff told the Messengers that the child, at this age, had a 30–50 percent chance of surviving but a 90 percent chance of developing intracranial bleeding if it survived, risking some degree of mental and physical handicap. The Messengers at that point instructed Dr. Karna that they did not want the baby resuscitated after birth or placed on intensive life support.
>
> Dr. Karna later stated that her reply to this instruction from the parents was something like, "Well, we'll see." She apparently felt that she had indicated to them that she was unwilling to consent to the nonresuscitation plan without at least evaluating the baby after birth. The Messengers, from their point of view, assumed that she had agreed with them not to resuscitate.
>
> At 11:38 p.m., Michael Messenger was delivered by cesarian section, weighing 1 pound, 11 ounces (770 grams). The infant was brought to the NICU and placed on a ventilator.
>
> At 12:10 a.m. Dr. Messenger went to the NICU and was surprised to learn that his son had been placed on intensive life support. At 12:40, Ms. Messenger arrived from the recovery room and the Messengers asked to be left alone with their son. Shortly after this request was granted, Dr. Messenger unhooked the ventilator. Alarms sounded but no NICU staff intervened to try to put the infant back on the ventilator and the baby died.[14]

After a bitter and extensive investigation, with hospital personnel deeply divided about the rightness or wrongness of Dr. Messenger's actions, the local district attorney charged Dr. Messenger with manslaughter. Thus, unlike most of the other NICU cases, which played out as either child abuse/custody battles or as malpractice cases, this one ended up in criminal court. In child abuse cases, the remedy is usually to take custody of the baby away from the parents. In malpractice cases, the plaintiff is seeking monetary compensation. In a criminal case, the jury is asked to decide whether the defendant should go to jail. For such a decision, the standards of evidence are quite different and the prosecutor must prove "beyond a reasonable doubt" that the defendant is guilty of the alleged criminal act. In the Messenger case, the jury eventually acquitted him of all charges. The case was not appealed. Given that it was a jury trial and that juries do not write opinions about their reasoning, it is hard to know just how the jury was thinking through the knotty issues of propriety, culpability, and legal accountability.

It is also interesting to examine this court's findings alongside the findings of the Texas Supreme Court in the Miller case and try to find some areas of overlap that might suggest consensus. Clearly, this was a baby who had some chance for survival, so by the Texas criteria, doctors were correct in not agreeing to a prenatal decision to withhold treatment. Instead, they appropriately insisted on their obligation to assess the newborn in the delivery room. That assessment then showed the baby to be vigorous and of a birthweight and gestational age that were both compatible with long-term survival. Thus, the approach taken by the doctors in overriding a parental request for nontreatment based on their assessment of the baby in the delivery room would have been upheld in Texas.

But they were not the ones on trial in Michigan. The real question is whether, after that initial assessment, a parent's decision to withdraw life support should be implemented. It is unclear what the doctors would have done had Dr. Messenger not discontinued his baby's ventilator but had asked them to do it. The way the case played out, these judgments could not be made and so cannot be evaluated. However, it seems clear today that a baby with a 50–50 chance of survival should probably be treated, at least until it is clear whether the baby will develop any of the admittedly imperfect but nevertheless informative clinical signs suggesting a bad outcome, such as a brain bleed, seizures, or prolonged ventilator dependence.

Perhaps the most interesting but least-publicized twist in the Messenger case came after his acquittal. A year later, Dr. Messenger sued the hospital and the doctors, claiming that the information that they had given him about the baby's chances for survival was misleadingly pessimistic and that if he had been given accurate information, he never would have disconnected his baby's ventilator. This lawsuit, which apparently never went to trial, is interesting for what it suggests about the process of communication and decision making.

Dr. Messenger thought that he understood the prognosis for his premature baby. As a physician, he was probably at least as well informed as an average parent. He made a decision based on his understanding at the time of the baby's delivery. Later, however, he came to realize that his knowledge was imperfect. He blamed the doctors for this misunderstanding.

A generous interpretation of the events of that day is not that the doctors were negligent but that, instead, communication at such moments of high stress is always imperfect. Doctors may not speak clearly; parents may not understand comprehensively, and the facts may be complex and change from minute to minute. These features of the situation are, in part, what led doctors to prefer a decision-making process that allows the irreversible decision of whether to withhold or withdraw life support to be made over a period of days, rather than minutes or hours. Doctors often suggest that parents go home and think about such a decision, discuss it with other family members, friends, or trusted advisers, and then reaffirm the decision. Such a process mitigates against decisions in the delivery room, at least in situations such as the one in the Messenger case, where treatment was not clearly futile.

Three cases from Wisconsin helped shape the way courts define the boundaries of physician obligations. In *McDonald v. Milleville*, Ms. MacDonald delivered an infant at 23 weeks of gestation. The baby weighed 600 grams. In the delivery room, Dr. Milleville initiated resuscitation measures. After 10 minutes of resuscitation, the infant's heart rate continued to be less than 50 beats per minute. Dr. Milleville discontinued resuscitation, told the parents that the baby was not viable, and suggested that they hold the baby until he died. One hour later, the infant began to cry. Examination showed that his heart rate was now above 100. He then received a full resuscitation and survived, though with severe neurological deficits.

The parents filed suit against the physician, claiming that his decision to stop resuscitation was negligent. They argued for two different domains of negligence. First, they claimed that his assessment that the baby was not viable and that further resuscitative efforts were futile was obviously wrong. Second, they claimed that they should have been consulted and allowed to participate in the decision to stop resuscitative efforts.

The jury cleared the doctor, suggesting that they understood both the limits of a physician's prognostic ability as well as the scope of the physician's professional expertise to make some clinical decisions unilaterally. This decision offers a different set of twists and turns than the Texas or Michigan cases on the process of evaluating appropriate decision making in the delivery room. Unlike those cases, these parents did not express their preferences about treatment. Instead, they seemed to trust the doctors to do the right thing. The doctor exercised the sort of clinical judgment that would, it seems, have been approved by the Texas court, deciding after assessing the newborn that further treatment was unlikely to be beneficial.

The case turned, as did the Messenger case, less on the appropriate standard for treatment than on the appropriate standard for communication. What, exactly, did the doctor have an obligation to communicate with the parents before making a medical decision of any kind? How completely must the decision to stop be a shared decision? One could argue that the doctor's telling the parents that resuscitation had failed and giving the parents their baby to hold was an opportune moment for the parents to have raised questions or concerns. They did not.

This case, like the Miller case, is also mysterious in that there were, apparently, no further discussions about withholding or withdrawing life-sustaining treatment after the baby was admitted to the NICU. It is hard to tell, from the case records, whether such discussions took place, in part because they were not the focus of the litigation and so were not relevant to the particular court proceedings. Again, this highlights the limitations of adversarial litigation as a policymaking tool.

A few years later, the Wisconsin Appellate Court heard a case similar to the Miller case in Texas.[15] The plaintiff, Nancy Montalvo, went into labor at 23½ weeks of gestation. After attempts to stop her labor failed, she and her husband, Brian Vila, signed an informed consent agreement for a Cesarean section. The baby, Emanuel, was born alive, resuscitated in the delivery room, and admitted to the NICU. Ms. Montalvo subsequently brought suit against both the obstetrician and the neonatologist for failure to obtain her informed consent for the treatment of Emanuel, stating that if she had known the long-term consequences of treatment and the risk of long-term disability, she would not have consented to the C-section or the subsequent resuscitation.

The court noted,

> The doctrine of informed consent comes into play only when there is a need to make a choice of available, viable alternatives. In the context of treatment required after the cesarean procedure was performed on Emanuel, there are two reasons why no available, viable alternative existed to give rise to the obligation to engage in the informed consent process . . . First, requiring the informed consent process here presumes that a right to decide not to resuscitate the newly born child or to withhold life-sustaining medical care actually existed. This premise is faulty . . . In Wisconsin, in the absence of a persistent vegetative state, the right of a parent to withhold life-sustaining treatment from a child does not exist. It is not disputed here that there was no evidence that Emanuel was in "a persistent vegetative state." Accordingly, the alternative of withholding life-sustaining treatment did not exist.[16]

The court went on, "The second reason why a viable alternate did not exist to trigger informed consent is the existence of the United States Child Abuse Protection and Treatment Act (CAPTA) of 1984 . . . The Act includes a provision preventing "the withholding of medically indicated treatment from a disabled infant with a life-threatening condition . . . The implied choice of withholding treatment, proposed by the plaintiffs, is exactly what CAPTA prohibits."[17]

Thus, the court argued, under the common law of Wisconsin and federal statutory law, Emanuel's parents did not have the right to withhold or withdraw immediate postnatal care from him. Thus, no viable alternative health treatment existed to trigger a requirement to begin the informed consent process.

Although the Wisconsin decision in this case differs from the Texas court's reasoning in *Miller* on some of the fine points of legal doctrine, such as the role of federal child abuse legislation, the conclusion has similar implications. Both courts suggest a process for decision making by which doctors make the decision about treatment in the delivery room after the baby is born, rather than having parents make the decision before the baby is born. If anything, the Wisconsin courts go farther, suggesting that both doctors and parents are bound by child abuse laws to continue treatment if the baby is alive and there is any chance of survival.

A third Wisconsin case (this one decided before the others) showed that there are some limits to its perception of this obligation. In the 1993 case of *Burks v. St. Joseph Hospital*, Shemika A. Burks (Burks) arrived at the emergency room of St. Joseph's Hospital in Milwaukee complaining of cramps and contractions. Burks was about 22 weeks pregnant and not expecting to deliver until August 10, 1993, almost 19 weeks later. One hour after she arrived, Burks gave birth to a baby daughter, Comelethaa, who weighed only 200 grams (approximately 7 ounces) and measured 11 inches long. The baby died at 10:15 a.m., 2½ hours after delivery. In a subsequent lawsuit against the hospital, Burks alleged that her daughter was breathing and had a heartbeat at birth. She claimed the hospital staff denied her requests for medical assistance to the infant after birth and that the baby died in her arms. These claims were dismissed, with a finding that nonresuscitation of a 200-gram baby, even a baby born alive with a heartbeat and respirations, was within the standard of care.

Two things are clear from reading these cases. First, because the law seeks generalizability at a level of abstract principles, it is a blunt instrument to use in regulating clinical decision making in individual cases. Second, the law is excellent in defining what is at stake, in articulating the principles, and in setting forth considerations that should guide decision makers.

One interesting feature of all these Wisconsin cases is that, like the Miller case, they all focus on decisions made at the time of birth. We could find no cases that arose from controversies about decisions later in the neonatal course. This is particularly interesting because it is abundantly clear that decisions are being made to withhold or withdraw treatment after the neonatal period. In our NICU, the frequency of do not resuscitate orders increased from 29 percent of deaths in 1988 to 56 percent of deaths in 1998. Other NICUs report similar trends, both in the United States[18] and in Europe.[19] The picture we get of NICU decision making from descriptive epidemiology looks very different from the one we get from case law. In most cases, decisions are reached that are not adversarial or confrontational. If our analysis of the process by which moral paradigms are applied in the NICU is correct, then the phenomenon of increasing numbers of decisions to withhold or withdraw life-sustaining treatment is appropriate. Doctors initiate treatment as a time-limited trial of therapy. This allows doctors to refine their prognostic estimates in a way that makes treatment withdrawal more individualized and thus more ethically defensible.

Overall, then, the picture that emerges from this legal and regulatory trend suggests that a rough consensus has developed. The thrust of legal maneuvering in the 1980s was to disempower doctors to make unilateral decisions based on quality-of-life assessments. The legal cases of the 1990s suggest that parents' rights to make unilateral decisions are also limited. There is widespread agreement that prenatal assessments of a newborn's viability or prognosis are always tentative. Doctors have the legal right to modify their prenatal assessment in the delivery room after they have had a chance to examine and assess the newborn baby. Thus, the law will not uphold parental rights to either demand treatment in situations where doctors think the baby is not viable nor parental rights to insist that treatment be withheld in the delivery room in situations in which doctors think the baby might do well. After that initial assessment is made, the law is much less well defined. Doctors and parents engage in a decision-making process that seems to take place well below the legal radar. Because these decisions have not been subject to legal scrutiny, the law remains largely undefined. Researchers are just now beginning to focus on these murkier domains of decision making.

THE MELDING OF CLINICAL AND LEGAL PARADIGMS: CONSENSUS ABOUT FACTS

The clinical facts and the legal constraints lead to fairly widespread consensus about NICU decisions. Decisions to withhold or withdraw life-sustaining treatment are permissible only when there is a low likelihood of survival or if survival is likely to accompany significant neurological or physical impairments. If those conditions are not met, treatment is morally and legally obligatory. Babies have rights to medical treatment that are independent of their parents' desires or their doctors' values.

The key, then, is to operationalize the abstract concepts of "a low likelihood of survival" or "significant impairment" to each particular clinical situation. The first cut on making this distinction in the NICU is the simplest one. As we have shown, birthweight is the strongest specific predictor of both morbidity and mortality in the NICU. Small babies are less likely to live and more likely to be impaired if they do survive than larger, more mature babies. Thus, there is, and has always been, some birthweight below which treatment has not been considered obligatory. The difficulty with this first cut is that the threshold for treatment itself has been changing over time. However, the gradual slowing of progress has led to some stability in consensus that governs current practice in the United States.

Today, babies who weigh more than 750 grams or who are born after 25 weeks of gestation have survival rates of 80 percent or more. Many of the survivors have no chronic health problems or only mild ones. This level of success precludes discretionary parental refusal of intervention.

At the other end of a relatively narrow spectrum of birthweight and gestational age, babies who weigh less than 400 grams or who are born before 22 weeks of gestation rarely survive. For these babies, then, treatment is rarely offered. Most neonatologists do not even attempt delivery-room resuscitation of infants who weigh less than 400 grams at birth.

Thus, the zone of birthweight-specific moral controversy and of parental discretion related to the treatment or nontreatment of their babies based on prematurity, is roughly between 400 and 750 grams, or between 22 and 25 weeks of gestation. Note, however, that these are criteria only for the initiation of treatment in the delivery room.

Many doctors view the initiation of treatment in the delivery room for tiny babies as the start of a "trial of therapy." Their hope is that the babies will "declare themselves." That is, they watch the babies closely over the first days of life to see whether the babies are developing conditions that are associated with a poor prognosis, such as intraventricular hemorrhage, severe lung disease, or sepsis. These criteria allow refinement of prognostic estimates, both in terms of survival and in terms of long-term chronic health problems or neurologic deficits. Ultimately, then, decisions for premature babies become less dependent on birthweight and are more driven by an individualized prognostic estimate.

A further refinement of prognosis takes place. Some of these babies develop conditions that make it seem as though death is inevitable and further treatment likely only prolongs the dying process. Such babies might, for example, have multisystem organ failure and worsen despite antibiotics, maximal ventilatory support, and vasopressors. In such clinical situations, decisions to withdraw life support are often seen as recognitions of the futility of further treatment rather than as attempts to avoid survival with poor quality of life. These are generally the least controversial decisions, even though, as we have shown, doctors may be wrong in their assessment that treatment is futile.

A second group of babies is more ethically controversial. They are the babies for whom survival is possible but for whom survival is likely to be accompanied by impairments of one sort or another that might be so severe as to make people question whether it is morally obligatory to prolong their lives. These might be babies with severe lung disease that makes them ventilator dependent; severe neurological damage leading to intractable seizures and profound mental retardation; short-gut syndrome, which can lead to lifelong dependence on parenteral nutrition, or other chronic conditions. The presence of these conditions preempts prematurity itself as the primary moral consideration. It also shifts the focus of the moral analysis from the likelihood of survival to the anticipated quality of life for survivors.

Quality of life thresholds are hard to define in an abstract way. Attempts to do so in the past have been inadequate or useless. However, case-based examples of quality of life that become paradigms for decisions have developed and have become more useful as guides. For example, Down syndrome is now a paradigm case of a quality of life in which it is no longer permissible to withhold or withdraw life-sustaining treatment. This chromosomal condition is associated with mild to moderate mental retardation. Forty years ago, parents were routinely offered the option of nontreatment for their babies with Down syndrome who required surgery. That standard has now changed. Down syndrome, today, is a paradigm case example of a condition in which treatment is considered obligatory. Thus, any case that seems analogous to Down syndrome is a case in which treatment withdrawal is not permissible.

An example of a paradigm case at the other extreme is anencephaly. This is a syndrome associated with complete absence of the cortex of the brain and is widely recognized as a syndrome that leads to a quality of life below the threshold at which treatment should be considered obligatory. For many people, anencephaly represents a paradigm case of medical futility. That is, they see it as a condition in which treatment is always inappropriate and ought never to be provided. At least one court decision, however, has opposed such an approach and instead allowed parental preferences to guide clinical decision making.[20]

Between Down syndrome and anencephaly, there are a number of syndromes that define the "gray zone." Other chromosomal anomalies, such as trisomy 18 or trisomy 13, lead to syndromes that cause severe mental retardation. They are also usually associated with congenital anomalies of the heart or other organs. These are syndromes in which it is permissible but not obligatory to withhold or withdraw life-sustaining treatment.

The relevant features of these three syndromes can be summarized. Down syndrome causes mild to moderate mental retardation. It is associated with both surgical and medical problems, but most of these problems can be successfully treated. Average life expectancy for individuals with Down syndrome is about 45 years.[21] Anencephaly is associated with mental impairment so severe that there is no chance of consciousness or awareness. Furthermore, few babies with the condition survive for more than a few weeks. Trisomy 13 and 18 cause severe mental retardation. Most babies with these chromosomal anomalies die within the first year, but 10 to 25 percent survive beyond their first birthday.[22] Survival is clearly associated with the decision to continue life support and the treatment of intercurrent illnesses. Thus, each of these three syndromes is associated with cognitive impairment and with shortened life expectancy of differing degrees. Either factor, by itself, if severe enough, would be enough to justify a decision to withhold or withdraw life-sustaining treatment. If neither factor is severe enough, then the decisions about the appropriateness of forgoing life-sustaining treatment rest on a complex algorithm that tries to incorporate both factors.

Such algorithms are necessarily inexact. They do not lead to rigid rules or to universal consistency. Instead, they reflect moral intuitions, cultural understandings, legal precedents, economic considerations, religious values and family dynamics. There are advantages and disadvantages to the inexactness of the criteria. Rigid criteria would avoid the stress of struggling to come to a decision, but would lock people into rules and regulations that may not reflect personal moral or spiritual values. Less rigid criteria allow moral discretion that sometimes leads to troublesome decisions. The tension between these two risks seems unavoidable and ineradicable. Ultimately, then, the freedom to make decisions within defined constraints shifts the focus from defining the zones of permissibility to understanding the process that takes places within the permissible zone.

THE MORAL PSYCHOLOGY OF DECISION MAKING

This discussion has focused largely on advances in clinical epidemiology. We have tried to summarize what neonatologists have learned about prognostication for VLBW babies. When the data are presented in this dry, empirical way, they suggest a process for decision making that is logical and ethically defensible as a way of maximizing the chances for intact survival for as many babies as possible. By this approach, doctors should initiate treatment in the delivery room for all babies over 500 grams birthweight. They should then reassess these babies frequently, looking for objective or subjective predictors of a bad outcome. Then, if such predictors are present, they should discuss with the parents the option of withdrawing life-sustaining treatment and allowing the baby to die.

This approach leads to some thorny and predictable emotional patterns. These result from the fact that this approach requires a decision to withdraw life-sustaining treatment, rather than a decision to withhold such treatment. Ethicists and legal scholars have always agreed that there is no moral or legal difference between *withholding* and *withdrawing* life-sustaining treatment. However, doctors, nurses, patients, and family members have always insisted that there are striking emotional differences between the two approaches to *forgoing* therapy. Put simply, it is much easier, emotionally, to withhold a treatment than it is to withdraw one.

This is illustrated in both empirical studies and in personal narratives. Empirical studies show that doctors generally find it emotionally less disturbing to withhold therapy than to withdraw it.[23] Furthermore, doctors prefer scenarios in which treatment withdrawal will lead to death relatively quickly to those in which the death process is more drawn out. Thus, they would rather withdraw ventilators or vasopressors than fluids or antibiotics.[24]

Parents seem to share these emotional preferences although the data on this are more scanty and anecdotal. In general, parents seem much more willing to opt for withholding treatment in the delivery room than they are to request or accede to withdrawal of life support for a baby in the NICU. This may reflect the growing emotional bond that forms between parents and their newborn, especially when the newborn is critically ill and extraordinarily vulnerable. Empirical studies of the emotional issues parents face in association with decisions to withdraw treatment are urgently needed. If they bear out the anecdotal experience of many pediatricians, they will suggest a complex dynamic by which it becomes increasingly difficult to withdraw treatments once they have started. Such an emotional pattern would create a powerful force that would challenge the usefulness of the epidemiological, ethical, and legal arguments for why treatment withdrawal after a "trial of therapy" is preferable to treatment withholding in the delivery room. Careful attention to this tension will likely become one of the big neonatal ethics issues over the next decades.

The decision to withdraw treatment is emotionally difficult for both professionals and parents. Some parents describe the decision as one in which they are asked to kill their own baby. However, many parents fear overtreatment and insist that they have the right to participate in decisions. In fact, much of the litigation surrounding end-of-life decision making in the NICU has been initiated by parents who felt that their consent for treatment was not sought, their views were not heard, and their preferences regarding treatment were not respected. Given this spectrum of parental response to the dilemmas, doctors must choose an approach of shared decision making.

Over the years, different schools of thought have evolved about the proper tone and structure for discussions about the withdrawal of life support. These might be characterized as the "objective information" approach, the "broad shoulders" approach, and the "shared deniability" approach.

In the objective approach, doctors try to give information to parents in the most nondirective way. Their goal is to educate, to give parents facts, and to empower parents to understand those facts. Such empowered parents are then free to come to a decision that reflects their own moral or spiritual values. In this approach, the doctor avoids making any recommendation about the appropriate course of treatment. If the parents ask the doctor what to do, the doctor ought to refuse to answer. In describing this approach, Truog writes, "when dealing with questions of value, physicians should see their role as facilitative rather then directive. Being nondirective, however, is not the same as being silent. An excellent model for this type of interaction is that of the psychotherapist. . . . Just as a good therapist would rarely, if ever, give a direct answer to the question, "Now tell me doctor, if you were me, would you divorce my wife?" so should pediatricians be reluctant to provide direct answers to similarly profound questions from parents. The job of the clinician in this case is to guide the patient or parent to a choice that is authentic and genuine for them."[25]

The moral psychology of this approach reflects a desire not to be coercive. It views doctors as disproportionately empowered and parents as thus problematically vulnerable to being overpowered by doctors' knowledge and authority. Given that sociological reality, proponents of this view argue that doctors have a moral obligation to err on the side of restraint. Sociologists who have examined the power structures of NICUs point out that such fears are valid and that the values of the doctors (or of the NICU culture more broadly) often dominate those of the parents. This occurs in both subtle and blatant ways. Philosophical support for this position comes from a respect for individual autonomy as the paramount moral principle.

This view has been challenged by those who point out the peculiarities of decision making in the context of critical illness. Such critics argue that medical decision making in these contexts is quite different from decision making in other contexts. Deciding whether to let one's baby die is not like deciding which minivan to buy, which college attend, or even whom to marry.

Two features of medical decision making highlight its uniqueness. First, medical decision making almost always takes place in the context of a unique relationship with a healer. Medical decisions take place in the context of the doctor-patient relationship. This relationship has been the focus of an enormous body of analytic literature over thousands of years. The existence of this special relationship itself testifies to the unique nature of the decisions that must be made. The need for a process of shared decision making derives from the enormous difference in the sophistication of the information that doctors have compared to patients. Knowledge of illness, treatment, prognosis, side effects and other factors is often quite complex and difficult to understand. Truly informed consent requires lengthy and difficult conversations. Many studies show that, even with such conversations, patients often do not understand key elements of their illness or of the proposed treatments.

The second unique component of decision making in the context of acute illness has been less well described philosophically but is often discussed in narrative descriptions by patients (or parents) who write about their own illnesses. In these accounts, illness seems to distort rationality in predictable and disturbing ways. Most people's thought processes change while they are in the midst of a health crisis. The emotional, spiritual, and physical stresses of illness make patients feel exhausted and vulnerable. People who are ill and suffering are in a different psychological and metaphysical state than healthy people. Literature by patients or about sickness suggests that they exaggerate fears, crave reassurance, eschew rationality, and deify their doctors.[26] Denial, magical thinking, and a focus on the present rather than the future are all expected, and perhaps desirable, responses to news of serious illness.[27]

Recognizing these unique features of illness, some have suggested that it is not enough for physicians to give objective information and to allow patients to then make decisions. Instead, doctors should try to understand as best they can the patients preferences, goals, and values, and then the doctor should make the decision for the parents. It should be the decision that the doctor thinks is most consistent with what the patient would want but may not be able to say. By this view, patients' (or parents of patients) particular vulnerabilities create a moral requirement for doctors to take some of the burden of decision making upon themselves. The image of "broad shoulders" captures this notion of medical responsibility. Instead of simply giving parents the facts and asking them to make a decision, doctors should make a recommendation.

In advocating this approach, Meyers writes, "Throughout most of their medical lives, patients are socialized to be heteronomous, rather than autonomous. Yet, at the worst possible time—critical care decision making—when life and death consequences are attached to the choices, the paradigm shifts and real consent is sought, even demanded, thereby making an often traumatic situation even harder."[28]

A third approach, the shared deniability approach, is harder to describe and perhaps more theoretical. It draws less on philosophical theory than it does on notions of spirituality and is seldom explicitly advocated but is often recounted in literary descriptions of decision making. We recently tried to explain this approach by analyzing novels by Dostoevsky and Oe.

Dosteovsky's *The Brothers Karamazov* is not explicitly about medicine, but it is about the group psychology of decision making within families. Furthermore, it focuses on a life-and-death decision.

The novel opens with a discussion of why the father, Fyodor Karamazov, does not deserve to live. He is an evil, nasty man, a drunk, a child abuser, a rapist, and a cheat. Three of the four sons clearly wish he were dead. It is unclear whether any of them will actually murder him, but they are clearly considering the idea. They talk and bluster, testing their moral sentiments about whether Fyodor deserves to live or die.

At one point, Dimitri, the oldest son, and Fyodor are having a particularly heated argument and Dimitri threatens to kill Fyodor. At the time, Ivan, another son, who is living in the house with Fyodor, is planning to go on a trip to Moscow. Smerdyakov, Ivan's half-brother, suggests that, if Ivan leaves, then Dimitri might kill Fyodor. His conversation is both a warning to Ivan and, in a subtle way, an encouragement. Although he suggests that Ivan's leaving might result in Fyodor's death, he nevertheless suggests that Ivan ought to go. Ivan is intrigued by Smerdyakov's seemingly mixed message. He tries to explicitly articulate what his half-brother is telling him. The conversation that follows suggests how hard it is to articulate such truths and how, instead, they are left somewhere beneath the surface of conversations, understood but perhaps never quite acknowledged. Ivan says,

> "Why on earth do you advise me to go . . .? If I go away, you see what will happen here." Ivan drew his breath with difficulty.
>
> "Precisely so," said Smerdyakov, softly and reasonably, watching Ivan intently.
>
> "What do you mean by 'precisely so'?" Ivan questioned him, restraining himself with difficulty.
>
> "I spoke because I felt sorry for you. If I were in your place I would simply give it all up . . ." answered Smerdyakov, with the most candid air looking at Ivan.
>
> "You seem to be a perfect idiot and what's more . . . an awful scoundrel." Ivan got up suddenly from the bench. He was about to pass through the gate, but stopped short and turned to Smerdyakov. He bit his lip, clenched his fists, and, in another minute,

would have flung himself on him. But Smerdyakov shrank back. The moment passed without harm to Smerdyakov, and Ivan turned in silence toward the gate.

"I am going to Moscow tomorrow, if you care to know, early tomorrow morning. That's all!" he suddenly said aloud in anger.

"That's the best thing you can do," Smerdyakov replied, as if he expected to hear it.[29]

Later in the novel, it becomes clear that Smerdyakov understood from this conversation that Ivan wanted his father killed. Smerdyakov not unreasonably thought that Ivan's decision to leave early the next morning was a clear and unambiguous sanction of Fyodor's murder. It is not clear what Ivan thought. The next morning, Ivan leaves for Moscow. That night, Fyodor is killed, just as Smerdyakov predicted. Dimitri is arrested and charged with the murder. The remaining two-thirds of the novel is an examination of guilt and accountability for the murder of Fyodor.

Such a fictional episode may seem to have little to do with informed consent, medical ethics, or decisions about withholding life-sustaining treatment in the NICU. However, Dostoevsky's story is about much more than one particularly dysfunctional nineteenth-century Russian family. It is about the motivations, the self-deceptions, the enigmatic conversations, the understandings and misunderstandings, the conversational gropings that flow in and around and through the words and silences that characterize family decision making around life and death issues. It is about the tension between a sinful act, on the one hand, and a tragic situation, on the other. In this sense, it is about the moral and psychological universe of the NICU or the PICU where, for most parents, the tension is not between right and wrong but is between sin and salvation, or between two different forms of wrong that are incomparable, incomprehensible, and irreconcilable. Is it better to authorize continued painful treatment of a baby who has little likelihood of survival and a high likelihood of ongoing misery even if they do survive or to authorize shamefully and cowardly the death of one's own baby? What sorts of rationality can help here? What sorts of supportive relationships? It seems that, for most parents, these are not decisions that can be reasoned through in ways that lead to logical conclusions. Instead, they are vast gaping rifts in the universe, miasmas of pain and tragedy where every choice is wrong, and the only options are for different kinds of lifelong guilt, suffering and remorse.

In the novel, the response to this sort of dilemma is to avoid explicit discussion. In fact, the closer Ivan and Smerdyakov got to explicitness or honesty about their feelings, thoughts, and motivations regarding Fyodor, the angrier they became and the more difficult it was for either of them to say precisely what they meant or felt or wanted. Whatever the brothers wanted, explicit conversation was not part of it. Throughout the novel, Dostoevsky makes the point that, although everybody wanted Fyodor to die, and many people even expressed a willingness to kill him, nobody wanted to take individual responsibility for the decision or the action.

Such sentiments, we believe, are similar to those of family members who are asked to make a decision to withhold or withdraw life-sustaining treatment. They may want the treatment to be withdrawn, but they often do not want to take responsibility for the decision. We recently interviewed doctors, nurses, and parents of babies who died in the NICU, asking them to describe the process of decision making. One doctor described the following scene,

> I talked to the parents about (stopping the ventilator). I told them we can't make their baby better and that we wanted withdraw support. Dad said, "You can't. That's murder." And then he clenched both hands and started to come towards me. I thought he might hit me, but he walked passed me and hit the wall. It was a strange moment. It's like time stood still. I watched him come towards me and I just stood there—I didn't want to flinch, because I didn't want him to think that I didn't trust him. And I wanted them to trust me. But I thought he might hit me. But fortunately he didn't and he didn't hurt anybody. He went out the door. A few minutes later, I saw him in the hall and he asked me if I had done it yet. I said I was on my way now. I turned off the oxygen and went up on the fentanyl to keep her comfortable. The father saw me and smiled. He was tearful and he left, smiling at me. It was a big turn around for him.[30]

One might ask whether this interaction led to a decision, and, if so, who made the decision. It seems that neither the doctor nor the father would or should take total responsibility but that, instead, each might feel both partial accountability and partial deniability. The father could say that the doctor forced the decision on him. The doctor could say that the father ultimately agreed to the decision. Both the Karamazovs and this father seem to arrive at their decisions without the willingness to admit that they were arriving at a decision. Instead, they deny their moral sentiments and condemn those with whom they are collaborating. They evade the central moral issues and give contradictory messages. They test the emotional waters with ambiguous expressions of complicity or rage to see whether their feelings will be met with tolerance or condemnation. Similarly, in the neonatal case, as in many cases in clinical situations, doctors, patients, and family members arrived at a decision in a way that allowed everybody to feel absolved of individual responsibility for the decision.

After such conversations, everybody is able to think that somebody else made the decision, that somebody else was morally accountable, that somebody else was to blame. A brilliant and sensitive description of this process appears in the novel, *A Personal Matter* by Nobel laureate Kenzaburo Oe. Oe creates a character named Bird whose newborn son is hospitalized with a severe congenital brain anomaly. The doctors have recommended surgery, even though they believe that surgery will likely leave Bird's son with severe neurologic deficits. One doctor described the likely outcome as "a vegetable existence." Bird does not want to authorize the surgery but also does not want to appear to be authorizing his son's death. The conversation between Bird and the doctor has a tone that is quite similar to the tone of the conversations described above, both assigning and avoiding responsibility:

> "No developments worth mentioning today. We'll have somebody from brain surgery examine the child in the next four or five days."
>
> "Then—there will be an operation?"
>
> "If the infant gets strong enough to withstand the surgery, yes." The doctor said, misinterpreting Bird's hesitation."
>
> "Is there any possibility that the baby will grow up normally even if he is operated on? At the hospital where he was born yesterday, they said the most we could hope for even with surgery was a kind of vegetable existence."
>
> "A vegetable—I don't know if I'd put it that way . . ." The doctor, without a direct reply to Bird's question, lapsed into silence.
>
> "You don't want the baby to have an operation and recover, partially recover anyway?"
>
> "Even with surgery, if the chances are very slight. . .that he'll grow up to be a normal baby . . ."
>
> "I suppose you realize that I can't take any direct steps to end the baby's life!"
>
> "Of course not—"
>
> "It's true that you're a young father—what, about my age." In a hushed voice that no one else on the ward could hear, he said, "Let's try regulating the baby's milk. We can even give him a sugar water substitute. We'll see how he does on that for a while."
>
> "Thank you," Bird said, with a dubious sigh.
>
> "Don't mention it."[31]

This dialogue is laced with double entendre, misunderstandings, hints and evasions. At certain points, the author leaves it ambiguous about which of the two characters is speaking. Nevertheless, they seem to reach a decision, but one that neither quite feels responsible for and one about which both are somewhat ashamed.

This approach to shared decision making is harder to defend philosophically than either the approach based on individual autonomy in which the doctors' role is to provide objective information or the broad-shoulders approach in which the doctor acts beneficently and paternalistically to shoulder the burdens of decision making. Both those approaches lead to a clear sense of accountability. We know who made the decision and who is to blame. The Dostoevskian approach, by contrast, has, as its goal, shared deniability. The ideal process of decision making is one in which nobody feels ultimately responsible and everybody feels that somebody else made the decision. This is a difficult goal to achieve because it rests on a sort of absolute ambiguity. Such ambiguity is, by its very nature, delicate and easily undermined.

CONSENSUS ABOUT PROCESS

These three philosophical approaches define a range of acceptable practice alternatives. Most doctors try to navigate a path somewhere among them. In doing so, they often follow a fairly standardized process.

Generally, when a baby is not doing well in the NICU, doctors initiate the process of decision making about the possibility of forgoing life-sustaining treatment by having a discussion with parents in which they try to explain the dire facts and the unattractive possibilities. Doctors rather than parents initiate most discussions about withholding or withdrawing life support for children in the NICU or the PICU. For example, in recent studies of such discussions in PICUs, parents initiated only 10 to 24 percent.[32] In a NICU study, doctors initiated 73 percent of such discussions.[33] Doctors lay out the possibilities for continued treatment or for nontreatment. They answer questions. Usually, this first discussion does not lead to a decision. Instead, it is adjourned and parents are allowed time to think. In most cases, they seek outside support—from extended family, from clergy, or from mental health professionals.

A second discussion usually follows within a few days in which a decision is reached. Three sorts of decisions can be reached. The first is that parents do not want to stop treatment and do not want to consider it in the future. They want "everything done" to keep their baby alive. Generally, this leads to a discussion of the ambiguity of the term "everything done" in today's medical environment. The second sort of decision that can be reached is a "time-limited trial" of continued treatment. By this approach, doctors agree to continue treatment for a defined period of time and to set certain parameters or end points that they might then look for to see whether the treatment is leading to anticipated goals. For example, doctors might offer to continue mechanical ventilation for another week and if, at that point, the ventilator can be safely discontinued, then it will be. If not, however, it will be discontinued anyway in a manner that will likely lead to the death of the baby. The final sort of decision that can be taken is a decision to withdraw life-sustaining treatment immediately. In those situations, there is a standard set of

NICU rituals that ensue. The staff in most NICUs is familiar with those rituals. The baby is moved to a separate room, the parents are present, the ventilator or the intravenous fluid pumps are removed, and the parents are allowed time alone to hold their dying baby.

These procedural approaches to decision making are not specified and are usually not understood as part of the moral evaluation of the decision-making process. They do, however, reflect at least three moral concerns. First, they reflect a delicate balance between the rights of parents to make decisions for their children and the obligations of doctors to make recommendations and share responsibility. We have come a long way from the 1970s, when some doctors felt that it was their obligation to make the decisions for parents, or when many parents perceived the professionals in the NICU as insensitive or hostile. Today, it seems, doctors and parents come together in a delicate dance of shared responsibility and accountability. Parents are ultimately responsible for the decision, but they are not solely accountable for it.

The second moral consideration that is reflected in this process is the need for careful consideration of options over time. Decisions are not made in a hasty way. Parents are encouraged to go home and think about options, to consult others, and to decide slowly. This is a way of testing the authenticity of the decisions. Decisions that are made hastily, especially in emotionally harrowing circumstances, may not be the best decisions. The deliberately slow process that characterizes most NICU decisions is designed to counter this trend.

Finally, the inclusion of other family members and other members of the family's community reflects a moral impulse to protect the family from isolation within their own emotional and moral community. It supports the notion that, for such decisions, it is often desirable to spread accountability widely, rather than focusing it narrowly. This may be the reflection of a desire for shared deniability.

In most cases, decisions to stop treatment are made by consensus. Thus, if consensus is not achieved, treatment continues. As a practical matter, this means that both doctors and parents have an effective veto power over decisions to withhold or withdraw treatment. This procedural need for consensus is the most frequent source of conflict, especially when either doctors or parents feel strongly that treatment should not be provided but they are unable to convince their decision-making partner. Parents in this situation sometimes sue. Doctors invoke medical futility as a moral trump card.

How well do these approaches work? It is difficult to know precisely how to measure quality or to evaluate outcomes in this area. We do, however, know a few relevant facts. First, the number of deaths in the NICU that follow a decision to withhold or withdraw treatment has been steadily increasing over time. In most NICUs today, over half the deaths are associated with such decisions.[34]

The current consensus leads to a balance of power between doctors and parents that is not always perceived as optimum. On the doctors' side, the most common objection to the current consensus arises in situations where they perceive parents as making unreasonable demands for the continuation of treatment in situations where the doctor perceives further treatment as futile. On the parents' side, the most common objection is in situations in which they fear the long-term sequelae of continued treatment but the doctors are not yet convinced that these potential sequelae justify discontinuation of treatment.

Further research might address the actual processes of coming to consensus and try to determine whether there are particular skills or techniques that facilitate the process. Such research might also characterize the difficulties that arise in the "trial of therapy" approach and quantify the phenomenon that many doctors allude to but that has seldom been rigorously studied of parental reticence to stop treatment increasing as time goes on. If this phenomenon is real, it might be better characterized through careful research.

Further research will probably also focus on the role of economics in the NICU, a zone of concern that has changed as much from the 1980s to the 1990s as have the moral standards, the clinical practices, and the law.

CHAPTER SIX

Economics of the NICU

The central question of NICU economics (and, perhaps, of all economics) is about comparative value. In economic terms, it might be phrased, "Is the product worth the cost?" With regard to NICUs, that question can be unpacked into a series of subtler questions. What, exactly, is the "product" of neonatal intensive care? How much does it really cost? Who will bear the cost? Who will benefit?

Questions of value arise in both economics and ethics. They can be analyzed with the tools of either domain of intellectual inquiry. Dollars have many real and metaphorical meanings. They are one of many ways that we have of reflecting the value that we assign to certain endeavors.

The simplest way to think about the product of neonatology is in terms of lives saved. In this approach, what we are buying when we spend money on NICUs is survival for babies who would have died otherwise. This measure is implicit in the assessments of the improvements in birthweight-specific survival rates that have been the benchmark of neonatology's success.

A modification of such an analysis tries to determine whether the amount of survival that we are buying is worth the cost. In this approach, we divide the incremental amount of life that has been saved by the total cost to obtain a measure of cost-effectiveness—dollars per life saved or dollars per year of life preserved.

A further modification of this technique adjusts overall survival rates by a factor that tries to take into consideration the chronic diseases or neurological impairments that afflict some survivors. These impairments are usually conceptualized as some detriment to the "quality of life." Overall survival rates are then transformed into "quality-adjusted" survival rates.

A different and more complex sort of economic analysis looks at the neonatal intensive care in the context of the complex market for health care in the United States. Within that market, health care products may thrive or wither not based on their overall cost or even, necessarily, their cost-effectiveness. Instead, survival is based on their profitability. Some health care interventions and technologies work quite well but are nevertheless not profitable, while others do not work well at all but nevertheless make money for those who purvey them.

In this chapter, we will analyze the NICU from each of these perspectives.

OVERALL COSTS OF NICU CARE

It is not easy to figure out exactly how much we spend on neonatal intensive care in the United States. Part of the reason for this is that the medical care of newborns is not covered by any single insurance source. In this, neonatology is distinguishable from geriatrics. For the elderly in America, Medicare is essentially the single payer. Thus, analyses of Medicare claims data can give reliable estimates of overall health expenditures. Either Medicaid or private insurance insures most premature babies. Unlike Medicare, Medicaid is administered by the states, so it is not a single payer but fifty-two (counting each state and the District of Columbia and Puerto Rico) different programs, each with its own rules and its own databases. Private insurance companies have no public reporting requirements. Thus, it is difficult to find or estimate summary statistics of national expenditures for neonatal care.

There is also some debate about which costs should be figured in assessing the cost of neonatal intensive care. Clearly, the costs of the initial NICU stay are crucial. However, many premature babies continue to generate health care costs and other costs long after they leave the NICU. For example, former preemies have five times the rate of hospitalization of full-term babies during the first year of life. Many former preemies require ongoing outpatient care from a variety of subspecialists. Some require complex home health care. NICU survivors with developmental problems may require ongoing physical, occupational, and speech therapy. They may require special education. It is not clear whether costs incurred by the school systems who must provide education for children with neurologic or cognitive problems ought to be considered health care costs, educational costs, social welfare costs, or be accounted for in some other way. Similarly, it is difficult to account for the costs to parents who leave work to care for their chronically ill children. These costs are even harder to estimate than the costs of the NICU care.

Even if all these costs could be calculated accurately, it is also not straightforward to decide which of these costs should be considered as costs of neonatology. After all, before neonatology existed, many newborns developed neurological problems or chronic diseases and required special education, repeated hospitalization, and home health care. Many of the babies who developed these problems in the pre-NICU era no longer do so. Therefore, an accurate economic analysis of these indirect costs would analyze the difference between costs today and the costs that would have been incurred by babies who would have developed neurologic problems in the absence of NICUs but did not. That analysis, of course, would be even more difficult.

Economists have tried to estimate all of these costs. Rogowski examined costs from 3288 admissions to a nationally representative sample of twenty-five NICUs in 1993–94.[1] She found that the average total cost per admission was about $50,000 (in 1994 constant dollars). For the smallest babies, those between 501 and 750 grams, the average cost was about $90,000. For babies between 1251 and 1500 grams, the cost was about $32,000. Table 2 shows the overall cost breakdown for VLBW babies in 1993–94 as calculated by Rogowski.

These numbers from twenty-five NICUs in the early 1990s allow us to estimate the total costs of NICU care in the United States. Overall, in the United States, there are about 250,000 admissions to NICUs annually. If the average cost is $50,000/baby, then a back-of-the-envelope calculation would put the direct cost of NICU care at about $12.5 billion in 1994 dollars. If we assume that the ratio of survivors to babies who die is about the same as in 1993–94 and that the number of NICU admissions is about the same, then these numbers would only need to be adjusted by health care inflation to determine the overall direct cost of NICU care today. Health care costs have gone up an average of 5.7 percent per year between 1994 and 2003.[2] Therefore, without other changes, the direct cost of NICUs in the United States in 2004 could be estimated at around $21 billion.

TABLE 2
Median Treatment Costs and Length of Stay for Infants with Very Low Birthweight

	N	Total Cost	Length of Stay	Cost/Day
All infants	3288	$49,457	49	$1,115
Birth weight				
501–750 g	601	$89,546	79	$1,483
751–1000 g	811	$78,455	72	$1,200
1001–1250 g	861	$49,097	49	$1,059
1251–1500 g	1015	$31,531	35	$ 932

Source: Reproduced with permission from *Pediatrics* 1999;103:329–35 Table 1. Copyright © 1999 by the American Academy of Pediatrics.

The indirect costs, including medical follow-up for secondary problems and social costs of disability among survivors, are more complex. A comprehensive recent review suggested that they are probably roughly equivalent to the direct costs.[3] Thus, they might also currently be between $15 and $20 billion. That makes the total cost of neonatal intensive care in the United States on the order of $25–$40 billion annually.[4] To put this number in perspective, overall national health expenditures in 1994 were about $950 billion.[5] They had risen to $1.6 trillion in 2002.[6] Thus, the initial and ongoing care of premature babies accounted for about 2 percent of national health expenditures. Some proportion of this expenditure is in the educational system, rather than the health system, so the true percentage of national *health* expenditures may be lower. If we just consider the direct costs for the initial NICU admission, the 250,000 babies who are admitted to NICUs annually are about 0.1 percent of the U.S. population and account for about 1 percent of national health care expenditures.

COST-EFFECTIVENESS OF NICUS

An analysis of the cost-effectiveness of NICUs tries to measure the dollars spent against some quantifiable outcome. Two quantifiable outcomes are commonly used: the total years of life saved, and "quality-adjusted" years of life saved. NICU care has been repeatedly analyzed in this way. In the early 1980s, Boyle and colleagues compared the cost-effectiveness of NICU care before and after a regionalized perinatal network was established.[7] They showed that "for newborns weighing 1000 to 1499 g, intensive care resulted in a net economic gain when figures were undiscounted but a net economic loss when future costs, effects, and earnings were discounted at 5 per cent per annum . . . By every measure of economic evaluation, the impact of neonatal intensive care was more favorable among infants weighing 1000 to 1499 g than among those weighing 500 to 999 g."

A study by Walker and colleagues analyzing data from the late 1970s came to similar conclusions. They showed that the costs/survivor were $363,000 for babies 600–699 grams, but only $41,000 for babies 900–999 grams. If one assumes that survivors live for 75 years, then the cost/year of life is about $4,800 for the tiniest babies and $600 for the bigger babies. Of course, as in the Boyle study, these numbers can be adjusted or discounted in a number of ways. They can also modified by considering quality of life. The authors of this study concluded that NICU care may not be cost-effective for the tiniest babies due to the high costs per survivor.

Thorny ethical problems arise with such an approach. These ethical problems were quantified in a 1988 study by Stoltz and McCormick.[8] They examined the economic and clinical effects that would result from policies that dictated withholding treatment from premature babies using various birthweight cutoffs. They looked at three specific cutoffs: 500, 600, and 700 grams. They showed that "policies denying care to infants born at <500, 600, or 700 g would lead to total NICU care savings of 0.8%, 3.2%, and 10.3%, respectively. Applying the local birthweight-specific survival rates, such policies applied nationally would not have offered care to 136, 575, and 2689 potential survivors annually. Birthweight-based rationing schemes also are shown to increase further the racial disparity of NICU deaths." In other words, cost-savings accrued only if treatments were denied to babies for whom the treatments were successful. These results are summarized in the Table 3.

More recent analyses of the cost-effectiveness of NICUs show that NICUs have become more cost-effective over the years between 1980 and 1997, primarily because they became more clinically effective. At each birthweight, there are more survivors, so more of the dollars that are spent are allocated to survivors. Thus, survival rates improve, overall costs of NICU care go up, but the overall cost per survivor stays relatively constant. Doyle and colleagues quantified this effect in Australia by comparing the 1970s, 1980s, and 1990s. They showed that "the cost-effectiveness ratios (expressed in Australian dollars for 1997) were similar between successive eras at 5270 dollars, 3130 dollars, and 4050 dollars per life-year gained, respectively. The cost-utility ratios were similar between successive eras at 5270 dollars, 3690 dollars, and 5850 dollars per quality-adjusted life-year gained, respectively, and were similar to the cost-effectiveness ratios."[9]

Cost-effectiveness studies might have nudged the field of neonatology in a different direction from the one that it ultimately took. To the extent that they suggested that there might be birthweight-specific cutoffs below which NICU care just wasn't worth it anymore, these economic calculations may have mapped onto clinical and emotional intuitions. Taken together, these two lines of reasoning might have led to guidelines that would pick some semiarbitrary birthweight cutoff—600, 700, or 750 grams—and say that NICU care will be provided only to ba-

TABLE 3
Potential Effects of Birthweight-Based Rationing:
Savings and Survivors at Varying Birthweight Cutoffs

Weight Cutoff (g)	NICU Savings	Survival Rate below Cutoff (%)	Annual U.S. Survivors Affected
500	0.8	0.15	136
600	0.2	0.20	575
700	10.3	0.38	2689
800	18.7	0.49	6126

Source: Reproduced and modified with permission from *Pediatrics* 1998;101(3):344–48, Table 2.
Copyright © 1998 by the American Academy of Pediatrics.

bies above that birthweight. This solution has been seriously considered, in the United States[10] as well as in England,[11] Sweden,[12] and Australia.[13]

This did not happen because of a different aspect of cost-effectiveness, one that we have tried to capture using a slightly different methodology.

We calculated the efficiency of neonatal care by looking at the overall number of bed days that were used by babies who ultimately went on to die, compared with the bed days used by babies who went on to survive. We found that most of the bed days, and thus most of the dollars, spent in the NICU go to survivors.[14] This is true regardless of the birthweight or gestational age of the baby. Even for the tiniest babies, more than 80 percent of the bed days were used by babies who ultimately survived.

We then compared the smallest babies in the NICU with the oldest adults in the medical intensive care unit (MICU). We found a sharp contrast. More than 80 percent of the bed days used for the sickest adults—those over 75 years of age and on a ventilator—were used by patients who went on to die. These results are shown in Figure 9. While cost-effectiveness comparisons are always complicated, these data suggested that by at least one crude measure—resources used on patients who would survive to leave the hospital rather than patients who would die before discharge-NICUs were much more efficient than MICUs.

This phenomenon entirely depends on the fact that dying babies die quickly. Some recent studies have suggested that this has changed over the past two decades and that babies who die tend to linger longer than they used to. For example, Hack and Fanaroff reported that the time to death for babies who died in their NICU increased dramatically throughout the 1980s.[15] Ellington and his group in Boston reported a similar increase in the length of time from admission until death for babies who died.[16] We have noted a similar phenomenon in our NICU—the median day of death for babies who died rose from 2 in 1991 to 10 in 2001.[17] Such increases in the length of stay for babies who are dying raise both ethical and economic concerns.

The ethical concerns have to do with the imposition of pain and suffering on babies and on families from the provision of futile care. The problem, of course, is in determining which care is futile for which babies. If we knew, on day 1, which babies were going to die on day 10, it would be much easier to justify withholding or withdrawing treatment from such babies. Because we do not know, we generally provide treatment to all babies. The gradual lengthening of the time period during which babies "declare themselves" ultimately results in a prolongation of the dying process for babies who ultimately die. Given prognostic uncertainty, a certain amount of such futile treatment seems inevitable. The alternative would be to withhold treatment from babies who might benefit to avoid treating babies who would not. This is not a trade-off that most parents or doctors are eager to make.

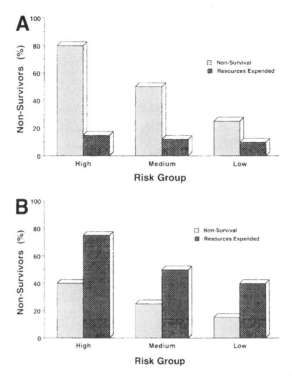

Figure 9 Bed days allocated to nonsurvivors in the neonatal intensive care unit and the intensive care unit. Reproduced with permission from Lantos JD, Mokalla M, and Meadow W. Resource allocation in neonatal and medical ICUs. Epidemiology and rationing at the extremes of life. *Am J Respir Crit Care Med* 1997;156:185–89. Copyright © Massachusetts Medical Society.

The economic problem is analogous. When most babies who were fated to die died early in their hospital course, NICU resources seemed to be used in a remarkably efficient manner. NICUs, much more than other ICUs, were able to target resources to patients who ultimately survived. To the extent that the dying process is prolonged, this may no longer be the case. To test whether this phenomenon has occurred, we examined data from our NICU from recent years and compared it with the data from ten years ago. We found that, at least in our NICU, the trend toward a longer time until death was balanced out by improvements in survival. Over the ten-year span, the percentage of overall NICU bed days (equivalent to percentage of overall NICU dollars) devoted to doomed infants remained roughly constant at 4 percent—never rising above 6 percent or falling below 1 percent. This is true at all birthweights. Nonsurvivors continue to occupy a minute fraction of NICU resources. Even today, more than 90 cents of each NICU dollar is spent on infants who will go home to their families.

These sorts of measures of cost-effectiveness take a societal-level view of the economics of NICU care. Such analyses may be useful to policymakers who are trying to decide how to allocate resources within the health care system. If it could be shown, for example, that NICU care overall was not cost-effective, then Medicaid programs might stop reimbursing doctors or hospitals for such care.

Interestingly, the economics of NICU care became inextricably intertwined with the legal and political aspects of NICU care. After the Baby Doe controversy, in which the federal government tried to mandate treatment of almost all newborns, it became difficult to imagine a public policy in the United States that would allow care to be systematically limited. Instead, the opposite happened. Public policies were enacted that generously reimbursed NICUs. This led to a different sort of economic calculus for NICUs, one that focuses not on overall societal expenditures and societal benefits but that instead looks at the fiscal realities of individual hospitals and the doctors who work there. In our decentralized health care system, these economic forces are much more powerful drivers of actual behavior than the theoretical calculations of societal costs and benefits.

NICUS AND HOSPITAL FINANCE

Data on the hospital finances and on the role of NICUs within hospitals are even more difficult to obtain than data on overall expenditures for neonatal care. Nevertheless, it is clear that hospital administrators consider these matters when making decisions about whether to create, support or expand their NICU services.

In the 1960s and 1970s, it was unclear whether or not NICUs would be profitable or costly for hospitals. They represented, after all, an unprecedented investment in personnel, equipment, and infrastructure for a group of patients, newborn babies, who had never before been the focus of expensive medical interventions. Many traditional insurance plans did not cover newborn care. It was unclear what the "market" would be for NICUs. Successful implementation of regionalization would be necessary for any NICU to maintain the census that it needed to cover the fixed costs, but it was unclear whether regionalization would succeed in this arena when it had failed in so many others.

By the 1980s, however, the answers to these questions had become much clearer. Regionalization was working. Insurance plans began to cover newborn intensive care. State Medicaid programs stepped up to pay for babies whose parents did not have health insurance. NICUs, surprisingly, became profit centers rather than cost centers. Gustaitis and Young studied the NICU at Stanford University in the early 1980s. They noted,

> For hospitals, the Intensive Care Nursery (ICN) constitutes one of the more lu-crative sources of income. The proportion of revenue earned for a hospital through neonatology is consistently higher than the proportion of licensed beds devoted to newborn intensive care. At the Stanford University Medical Center, in 1984, the cost per day for an ICN bed was $1550. The hospital had 663 licensed beds, 25 of which, or 3.7 percent, were designated for newborn intensive care. In fiscal 1982–3, revenues from the ICN were $9.47 million, 4.4 percent of a total $217.57 million in hospital rev-enues. In 1983–4, the amount rose to $11.09 million, or 4.7% of total revenues of $236.44 million.[18]

In addition, they note that 82 percent of the faculty-generated income for pa-tient care in the Department of Pediatrics came through the NICU (or ICN). The entire department shared this windfall. Thus, by the early 1980s, the NICU was sub-sidizing both the Pediatrics department and, to a certain extent, the entire hospital.

This role for NICUs in the internal economy of academic medical centers has continued. In part, this is because NICUs are one of the few areas of pediatrics in which inpatient activity is increasing rather than decreasing.

Outside the NICU, the number of inpatient days for children has been falling steadily and rapidly over the past twenty years. In 1980, children (excluding infants) ac-counted for nearly 9 million bed days. By 1993, that number was less than 6 million.[19]

This large drop in non-NICU hospital days for children is due largely to improve-ments in care. More diseases are preventable, through effective immunization pro-grams, than were twenty years ago. Improved outpatient care of patients with asthma,[20] diabetes,[21] and those in need of minor surgery[22] has led to more outpa-tient care, less inpatient care, and fewer hospital stays.[23] It has also led to a decrease in the length of inpatient stays for many illnesses.[24]

At the same time, the number of inpatient days in the NICU has been steadily rising. This is primarily because survival rates for the tiniest babies are improving. Those babies tend to have the longest NICU stays.

This phenomenon can be quantified. Nationally, there are approximately 53,000 babies born per year with a birth weight of <1500 grams. Survivors in this birth-weight group have an average hospital stay of nearly two months. Babies who die have shorter hospital stays. Thus, as overall survival rates improve, the total number of bed days used by these babies goes up. Overall, at today's survival rates, these babies account for 2.1 million bed days annually in the United States. Just a decade ago, when survival rates for such babies were lower, the bed days that they required were correspondingly fewer.[25]

The trend toward shorter inpatient stays for most children and longer inpatient stays for premature babies has implications for the economic survival of children's hospitals. Counting both NICU and post-NICU hospitalizations, neonatal intensive care units, and the care of chronically ill NICU survivors account for nearly half of the bed days in tertiary care children's hospitals in the United States today. The NICU has become the economic engine that keeps our children's hospitals running. The survival of hospital-based pediatrics as we know it is increasingly dependent on continued commitment to the technologies and the personnel that enable the survival of extremely premature babies.

At the University of Chicago Hospitals (UCH), the financial numbers are probably similar to those at other large hospitals around the country. In 2002, UCH had 25,500 total admissions, including adults and children. Of these, about 1000 (4%) were NICU admissions. The hospital had gross revenues of $525 million. Two-thirds of this came from inpatient care. Of the inpatient revenue, 10 percent came from the NICU. Thus, the NICU, which accounted for 4 percent of the patients in the hospital, generated 10 percent of the hospital's revenue.

By contrast, adult medical/surgical patients comprised 54 percent of admissions and 53 percent of revenue, adult cardiology patients comprised 10 percent of admissions and 11 percent of revenue, obstetrics had 15 percent of admissions and only 6 percent of revenue.

Put another way, the total operating margin of UCH in that year was $23.8 million. Of that, $11.4 million, or 48 percent, came from the NICU.

These sorts of numbers have an interesting effect on hospitals' strategic planning. Many hospitals are now building or expanding their NICUs in the hope that they will benefit from the profitability of NICUs. At UCH, a new children's hospital, opened in 2005. It has 10 percent more NICU beds than the old hospital.

A series of articles in the *Boston Business Journal* suggests the administrative dynamic at work. On August 30, 2002, the journal reported that a local hospital, the South Shore Hospital, had its bond rating downgraded "due to the hospital's declining operating performance."[26] On November 20, 2002, the journal announced that South Shore hospital was building a 10-bed NICU, making it the first nonteaching hospital in the state to do so.[27]

NICU ECONOMICS AND THE FUTURE
OF PERINATAL REGIONALIZATION

Interestingly, these economic forces have begun to undermine the perinatal regionalization programs that were so instrumental to the successful development of neonatology in the 1970s and 1980s (and to its current profitability). Howell and colleagues recently studied the extent of deregionalization of perinatal care in urban areas.[28] They showed that the growth of NICU beds has outpaced the need. "During the study period (1980–95), the number of hospitals grew by 99%, the number of NICU beds by 138%, and the number of neonatologists by 268%. In contrast, the growth in needed bed days was only 84%. Of greater concern, the number of beds in small NICU facilities continues to grow." Their data are summarized in the Table 4.

Is this proliferation of NICUs and NICU beds a problem? One can imagine two sorts of questions that might arise—one concerning clinical outcomes for babies and the other concerning the overall cost-effectiveness of NICUs. From a clinical perspective, the problem would be if babies at smaller NICUs had worse outcomes than those at larger, more traditional regional referral centers. The data on this are mixed. Multiple studies between roughly 1980 and 1995 were published comparing outcomes for infants cared for at level 3 units, compared with level 2 units. Indeed,

TABLE 4
Trends in NICU Hospitals, NICU Beds,
and Neonatologists, U.S. Metropolitan Statistical Areas, 1980–1995

	1980	1995	Change
Births, thousands	2729	3210	+18%
No. of hospitals with obstetric beds and children's hospitals	2135	1810	−15
No. of hospitals with NICU beds	351	698	+99
Obstetric/children's hospitals with NICUs, %	17	39	+130
No. of NICU beds	7021	16,702	+138
No. of neonatologists	710	2613	+268
NICU beds per 1000 births	2.57	5.20	+102
Neonatologists per 1000 births	0.26	0.81	+211
Occupancy rate of NICUs	76	78	+3
Total no. of hospital births, thousands	2729	3210	+17.6
No. weighing <1500 g	31,383	43,335	+38.1
% weighing <1500 g	1.15	1.35	+17.4
Total needed NICU bed days for infants weighing <1500 g	1.30 m	2.39 m	+83.8
Available bed days	2.56 m	6.10 m	+138.3

Source: Reproduced with permission, Howell EM, Richardson D, Ginsburg P, and Foot B. Deregionalization of neonatal intensive care in urban areas. *Am J Public Health* January 2002 92(1):119–24, Table 1.
Copyright © 2003 by the American Public Health Association.

one of the first practical applications of SNAP scores in neonatology was to analyze survival data across NICU centers, normalizing for illness severity of the inpatient population. When these analyses were performed, a consistent advantage to
inpatient care at level 3 centers was demonstrated.

For example, Cifuentes and colleagues reviewed mortality statistics for low
birthweight babies in California in 1992–93.[29] They showed that babies born in hospitals with regional NICUs had better survival rates. Interestingly, they did not use
the distinctions between level 1, 2, and 3 NICUs that have been the standard ways of
describing units in most perinatal regionalization programs. Instead, they used four
levels, which they characterized as no NICU / no intensive care, intermediate
NICU / intermediate intensive care, community NICU / expanded intermediate
intensive care, and regional NICU / tertiary intensive care. They found the biggest
differences between the first two categories and the latter two, with no differences
apparent between the later two themselves.

This idiosyncratic characterization of NICUs suggests that the evolution of regionalization has become quite complex. During the era between roughly 1982 and
1992, neonatology was rapidly advancing, and level 3 centers, mostly academic medical
centers, had access to a lot of things that level 2 centers did not—surfactants, in-house
neonatologists or neonatal fellows, neonatal nurse-practitioners, antenatal steroids,
oscillating ventilators, inhaled nitric oxide, and extracorporeal membrane oxygenation
(ECMO) to name just a few. So direct comparisons of outcomes for babies of similar
birthweights / gestational ages were likely to demonstrate a significant advantage for
the level 3 centers, and they did. Almost no study of that era compared level 2 versus
level 3 outcomes while controlling for equal access to these state-of-the-art techniques
and personnel. And there was no need to. The defining feature of the NICU level was
the availability of such professionals and such technology.

Today, we are in a different place. There is no current-day analogue to surfactant, an effective technology restricted to level 3 but not level 2 centers. Today, as
more and more neonatology fellows are trained each year, professional expertise is
no longer confined to level 3 centers. There are many more well-trained NICU
nurses and neonatal nurse-practitioners than the level 3 centers can accommodate.
The technology (monitors, ventilators, ultrasounds) is getting easier and more
user-friendly with each passing year. Thus, it would seem as if regionalization may
be an idea whose time has passed. If so, then neonatology will look more and more
like almost every other profitable and technology-intensive medical endeavor. It
will not be confined to designated referral centers. The monetary rewards for having a NICU will drive this transition. Consequently, regionalization qua central-
ization is a rearguard action. Eventually, and in many regions currently, a broad

acceptance of level 2 management of "stable" ventilated 1500-, 1250-, or even 1000-gram babies will be the norm.[30]

If the data were clear that deregionalization led to worse outcomes, then the moral and political pressure to maintain strict regionalization policies would be strong. Given the ambiguity of the data, however, it is easy to conclude that, if the outcomes are just as good and the costs of care are lower, then deregionalization would seem to be a good thing—no loss in quality, improved access, and cost savings.

When the level of analysis shifts back from micro to macro, however, the picture changes once again. Some recent research suggests that the proliferation of NICUs in the United States, driven by their profitability, is leading to profligate overuse of NICU technology. These data come from international comparisons. Thompson and colleagues examined this recently and showed that the United States has more neonatologists than other countries, "The United States has . . . 6.1 neonatologists per 10 000 live births; Australia, 3.7; Canada, 3.3; and the United Kingdom, 2.7. For intensive care beds, the United States has 3.3 per 10 000 live births; Australia and Canada, 2.6; and the United Kingdom, 0.67." These authors went on to examine whether this increased capacity led to better outcomes. Their disturbing conclusions were that "greater neonatal intensive care resources were not consistently associated with lower birth weight-specific mortality. The relative risk (United States as reference) of neonatal mortality for infants $<$1000 g was 0.84 for Australia, 1.12 for Canada, and 0.99 for the United Kingdom; for 1000 to 2499 g infants, the relative risk was 0.97 for Australia, 1.26 for Canada, and 0.95 for the United Kingdom."[31]

From a policy perspective, the solution to the problem of this problem of oversupply is straightforward; stronger regulation could eliminate smaller NICUs or at least make it less profitable for a small hospital to build and operate a NICU. From the perspective of each hospital, however, such regulation would interfere with their freedom to do business. Because NICU care has become a vital profit center for most academic medical centers, hospitals may favor such regulation, not because it is good for babies but because it is good for hospitals. Any change in policies regarding treatment or nontreatment will need to consider the financial implications within academic medicine, for nonacademic hospitals, and for health care systems as a whole.

Many countries in Europe have different mechanisms for funding neonatal intensive care. They also have different prevailing ethical norms. These may be related. For example, in the Netherlands, premature babies are much less likely to be intubated or placed on mechanical ventilation.[32] In a system of global budgeting, under which hospitals are not reimbursed more for providing more services, the economic incentives for the health care system as a whole and the economic incentives for each individual hospital are aligned. Lowering the total number of ventilator days, say, would free up hospital resources for other uses. In a system like the one in the United States, however, it would have the opposite effect. It would drastically lower hospital revenues and might prevent expenditures on other, less-profitable programs.[33]

THE CONVERGENCE OF ETHICS AND ECONOMICS

The development of an economic framework for NICU can be seen as a series of value choices that paralleled those made in the domains of clinical innovation, epidemiological evaluation, legal oversight, and moral evaluation. In each area, clear areas of widespread consensus have developed, along with areas of continued controversy. The areas of consensus are clear. First, the success of neonatology seems to be widely understood and broadly supported. This has led to a system of economic supports for NICUs that essentially make access to neonatal intensive care a right for every baby born in the United States and most developed countries without regard to the parents' insurance status or ability to pay. This reflects the uncontroversial medical success of neonatal care. Neonatology saves lives. In the United States as well as throughout the world, this success creates a moral, political, and economic imperative to find a way to provide such care to all babies who will benefit.

Such a broad political mandate, with its resultant permissive economics, creates financial incentives for overtreatment, rather than undertreatment. As hospitals become dependent on the profitability of their NICUs, fiscal considerations may tip the scale in situations where purely moral considerations would leave doctors and parents undecided. It is difficult to disentangle the strands of these intertwined considerations.

For the present, in the United States, it seems that the incentives are all aligned. Doctors want to provide more treatment. Society is willing to pay for it. Parents, in most cases, approve of it. And, in most cases, the treatment is beneficial. It seems to be all good. In the next chapter, we will examine some alternative approaches to the moral dilemmas that arise in the NICU.

CHAPTER SEVEN

Four Discarded Moral Choices

This book recounts and analyzes the complex, forty-year-long process by which moral consensus developed in the United States about certain aspects of neonatology. The complexity of the process reflects the nature of the problems. They were problems that touched areas of human existence, such as pregnancy, birth, and the intensive medical care of newborn babies, that had never before been the subject of such intense medical intervention. In the past, when there were no interventions to prevent the tragedy of an infant's death, there were no complex moral or medical decisions to be made. Medical interventions made it possible to avert such deaths and raised complex issues that required careful analysis. At the outset, neither the scope of the problems nor the domains of analysis were clear. The problems touched on domains of inquiry that were legal, medical, moral, political, economic, spiritual, and anthropological.

The resulting discourse about these matters thus included scholars in fields as diverse as moral philosophy, law, literature, economics, disability studies, epidemiology, psychology, communication studies, theology, sociology, political science, and anthropology. It also engaged families, journalists, filmmakers, and novelists. Across disciplines and modes of discourse, people wrestled with the issues, debated with each other, proposed solutions, critiqued such proposals, compromised, and sometimes came to wary and tentative areas of agreement.

Some but not all of these areas of conceptual or theoretical agreement were then translated into practical policies that guided the decisions and actions of doctors, nurses, and parents in NICUs around the country. Studies of the knowledge, attitudes, and beliefs of professionals and parents shed light on the degree to which they share the current consensus, the frequency with which they act in concert with it, and the ways in which they diverge from it. These studies, in turn, became grist for further analysis, part of the ongoing process of creating and refining a wholly new zone of moral thought and behavior. Taken together, this process has been one by which we, as a society, have come to a new understanding of ourselves and our moral obligations that is quite different from the understanding of those moral obligations that we started with decades ago.

It is easy to underestimate the significance of what has been achieved through this process. It is easy to say that not much has really changed and that the ethical debates today sound much like the ethical debates that took place decades ago. After all, this new consensus that we have today is not a new discovery or a break-through in knowledge. We didn't discover some radical new moral truth that we did not know before, akin to the discovery of the structure of DNA or a new vac-cine against polio. It is easy to find writings from the earliest days of neonatology that articulate moral values not dissimilar from the ones that are widespread today and to conclude that we are actually at the same place now as we were then. This view would be a misunderstanding of recent history and an underestimation of the work that it takes for society to respond to a new moral dilemma.

A moral breakthrough comes from a process of sifting through alternative moral arguments and trying to understand how they apply to new facts and new technologies. The process necessarily includes attentiveness to the political and economic implications of these developments. To be morally inclusive and politi-cally viable, the process must allow policymakers to listen in new ways to minority voices or voices that had not previously been heard. At the end, the process must propose a moral stance that tries to do justice to all these considerations. Remark-ably, all that has happened in neonatal bioethics.

The resulting consensus is a compromise. The nature of the process is such that no one internally consistent moral point of view prevails. Instead, the current con-sensus tries to take the most strongly held principles of each of the many con-stituents who have a stake in the outcome and to include as much as possible of as many as possible.

The present consensus is subject to change. It should be read less as the simul-taneous solution of a number of complex moral equations and more as analogous to a regression equation in statistics by which the best line is fit to data that are not strictly linear. New data will change the slope and position of the line. Such con-sensus building regarding moral values in new domains of human activity must be, by its nature, somewhat subtle, tentative, conditional, and modifiable. It is hard to know whether we have found the right balance, the best reflective equilibrium, the most stable compromises.

Some see the present consensus as inadequate or some aspects of it as morally reprehensible. For example, some people argue that parents' rights are unacceptably violated by the way that the current approach focuses on the independent rights of the baby. Others think that we spend far too much money on neonatal intensive care and that a more just and efficient allocation of resources would demand that we spend more on prevention. Some view all of neonatology is a vast medical experiment being conducted without appropriate institutional review or oversight, without the consent of the research subjects, and without the use of appropriate research methodologies. Such criticisms suggest that the process has been the opposite of progress and that instead we have been drifting rapidly in the wrong direction.

Oddly, both the view that we have made progress and the view that we are way off course are compatible with the central argument of this book. Such endorsements and critiques are an essential part of the ongoing process we describe. It is not necessary to support current practices in their entirety to recognize that a serious effort of moral reflection and analysis has yielded an equally serious collective work of moral synthesis. Because of that work, the moral landscape of neonatology has shifted over the past four decades.

Perhaps one of the best ways to understand just how this remarkable process works is to recognize some of the roads not taken, the moral options that were considered and then rejected, and to understand the process by which they were rejected. At least four such moral views can be articulated: (1) that we should spend more on the prevention of prematurity than we do and that, as a result, we will not have to spend as much on crisis intervention; (2) that NICU care for the tiniest babies is not worth the effort because of the unacceptably high rates of neurodevelopmental problems among survivors; (3) that parents alone should have the ultimate right to make decisions about treatment or nontreatment; and (4) that because all life is sacred, we must never discontinue life-sustaining treatment (or, in a somewhat softer version, that we should do so only in the narrowest of circumstances for the most severely impaired babies). We will examine each of these views and try to understand the grounds for its rejection as part of the public moral mandate.

Discarded moral view 1: Preventive care is morally preferable to NICU care because it is both cheaper and more effective.

One of the original stimuli for the development of neonatology was the concern that the infant mortality rate in the United States was unacceptably high.[1] In the early 1960s, as it became clear that the United States was slipping behind other countries in infant mortality rates, President Kennedy called for initiatives to lower infant mortality.[2] At this time, it appeared that there were two radically different approaches to the problem of infant mortality. One was to lower birthweight-specific infant mortality. The other was to lower the overall incidence of low birthweight. The former led in the direction of neonatal intensive care. The latter led more toward comprehensive preventive programs, including prenatal care. It was unclear which of these would be more successful or more cost-effective.

Part of the problem in assessing the relative costs, benefits, and utilities of the two different approaches is that they required very different delivery systems with very different funding mechanisms. Neonatal intensive care is a hospital-based system requiring significant up-front investment in personnel and equipment. NICUs then provide services to a relatively small number of children. By contrast, preventive prenatal care is a low-tech intervention that does not cost much for each individual case. However, because it is provided to so many more people, the overall costs are quite high. It is provided in the outpatient setting, not in hospitals. It must be provided to large populations of patients in the hope that it will prevent the need for costly hospitalizations in some small fraction of those patients. In general, hospitalization is paid for using health insurance reimbursement mechanisms (whether public or private). Preventive treatments, by contrast, are often not covered by insurance (at least before managed care) and are paid for either out-of-pocket or with public health dollars. Because of these different funding mechanisms, the overall costs are just one aspect of the financial puzzle. Decisions also reflect considerations about who will pay and who stands to profit or lose by the provision of services.

Throughout the 1970s, many people argued that the efficacy of neonatal intensive care had not been proved and that the efficacy of prenatal care was easily demonstrable. So, for example, Sinclair and colleagues wrote of neonatal intensive care programs, "The costs of neonatal intensive care are very high, and efficiency analyses comparing the costs and outcomes of intensive care programs and alternative programs will be required, if we are to continue to justify the existence and expansion of neonatal-intensive-care programs."[3] In this framing, the efficacy of "alternative programs" seems to be taken for granted or assumed.

Similarly, Silverman suggested that neonatology was on a misguided and politically dicey mission, "It is slowly dawning on the public that unrestrained intensive care of the smallest and the most seriously malformed neonates is unreviewed and unlegislated social policy. For example, how much of its resources should the community invest in social interventions to prevent premature birth, and how much in medical rescue in neonatal intensive care?"[4] Along these same lines, Kliegman talked about the "perinatal paradox" of better neonatal care with worse overall outcomes for children, "Despite the marvelous advances that permit us to treat respiratory distress syndrome, the continuing high low-birthweight rate places a significant strain on our health care system. The goal should be redirected to identifying large population-based efforts to reduce the number of low-birthweight infants."[5]

Based in part on these sorts of sentiments, a number of researchers did studies on the cost-effectiveness of programs to prevent low birthweight. In particular, they examined the efficacy of comprehensive prenatal care. In 1985, the Institute of Medicine issued a report called "Preventing Low Birthweight" that became the source for many future analyses of prenatal care programs. The IOM report concluded that "the birth of infants weighing less that 2500 g, and particularly those of 1500 g or less, imposes a large economic burden on our nation by contributing substantially to neonatal mortality, to disability among surviving infants, and to the cost of health care. The provision of adequate prenatal services, as currently practiced, to all pregnant women who receive public assistance and who have attained less that a high school education would require increased expenditures, but would decrease the overall fiscal outlays of governmental agencies for the care of the low birthweight infants born to these high risk women." Specifically, they concluded that the provision of comprehensive prenatal care would save the nation between nearly $30 million per year.[6] A report by the Office of Technology Assessment that reviewed fifty-five different studies came to the similar conclusion that low birthweight and neonatal mortality could be reduced if more pregnant women have early "comprehensive" prenatal care.[7]

Such analyses led to bipartisan support for federal Medicaid reforms that greatly expanded access to prenatal care. Republican Governor Michael N. Castle of Delaware summed up the prevailing sentiment, "Investing in your children is like compound interest—the benefits, in reduced costs to society, accrue year after year." And Senator Lawton Chiles said, "It is not often that a person in public life gets to say, 'I know how to save the lives of American children and save taxpayer money at the same time.' "[8] By the late 1980s, these ideas had become the conventional wisdom of the day. Led by the Bush-Quayle administration, there was bipartisan support for Medicaid expansions. At the press conference announcing the Medicaid expansion bill, liberal Democrats Henry Waxman and Bill Bradley joined conservative Republicans Henry J. Hyde and Mickey Leland to take credit for the legislation. All of this seemed relatively uncontroversial, politically appealing, and likely to be good for children.

The only problem with this politically appealing approach was that it turned out to be just plain wrong. This became clear as more careful analysis and well-designed demonstration programs were undertaken. In November, 1994, Huntington and Connell published a controversial paper in the *New England Journal of Medicine* entitled "For Every Dollar Spent—The Cost Savings Argument for Prenatal Care."[9] They examined in detail many of the studies that purported to show the effectiveness of prenatal care in reducing the incidence of low birthweight. They found a slew of serious methodological problems. These problems included the underestimation of the costs of prenatal care itself, underestimating the costs of overcoming nonfinancial barriers to access, and inaccuracies in determining both the real costs of postnatal care and the incremental costs if more high-risk mothers were to get into comprehensive prenatal care programs. Taken together, they argued, these methodological problems led to a misleading oversimplification of the relation between changes in the frequency of low birthweight and actual cost savings. They were at pains to point out that they were not against prenatal care as such. Instead, they were against the use of bad science for political ends, even if the ends were good ones. They argued that, "Rigorous evidence and a broad analysis are important, not only for the selling of this policy but also for the acceptance of future public health initiatives. Because the cost-savings argument has dominated the discussion, publicly funded prenatal care may abandoned if it turns out not to pay for itself."

Around the same time, studies began to appear that brought into question not just the assumption that prenatal care saved money but even that prenatal care would reduce low birthweight. Two types of analyses were done in this area. One looked at overall expenditures on maternal and child health and tried to correlate them with rates of low birthweight births. Becker and Teutsch analyzed data from states on expenditures and low birthweight rates. They write,

> Using expenditure data from the Public Health Foundation and National Center for Health Statistics, we compare the 10 states with the highest and lowest rates of low birthweight infants in 1980 and the 10 states with the most improved and least improved low birthweight rates over a 10-year period. We hypothesize that the 10 states with the best low birthweight rates and 10 states with the most improvement in low birthweight rates will be the states with the highest levels of maternal and child health expenditures per birth. We find *no support* (emphasis added) for the hypothesis in either group of states. At the state level, maternal and child public health expenditures do not appear correlated with states that are the most successful or are making the most improvement in low birthweight infants.[10]

The other type of study tried to understand the efficacy of comprehensive prenatal care programs in the highest-risk populations. Lu and colleagues recently published a systematic review of these data. They examined "original research, systematic reviews, meta-analyses and commentaries for evidence of effectiveness of the three core components of prenatal care—risk assessment, health promotion, and medical and psychosocial interventions—for preventing the two constituents of LBW: preterm birth and intrauterine growth restriction (IUGR)." After careful examination of the evidence, they show that, of all the interventions commonly associated with preventive prenatal care, only smoking-cessation programs were even modestly effective. Their pessimistic conclusion is that "neither preterm birth nor IUGR can be effectively prevented by prenatal care in its present form. Preventing LBW will require reconceptualization of prenatal care as part of a longitudinally and contextually integrated strategy to promote optimal development of women's reproductive health not only during pregnancy, but over the life course."

Overall statistics for the use of prenatal care and the incidence of low birthweight in the United States seems to reflect these epidemiological realities rather than the political myths that grew up around the flawed epidemiological studies of the 1980s. In 1984, 73 percent of pregnant women in the United States received prenatal care in the first trimester and the rate of low birthweight was 6.7 percent. Over the next twenty years, the percentage of women who received timely prenatal care steadily increased—to 76 percent in 1986, 81 percent in 1994, and 84 percent in 2002. At the same time, the percentage of babies born at less than 2500 grams birthweight increased to 7.3 percent in 1994 and 7.8 percent in 2002.

The fact that increased access to prenatal care did not reduce the percentage of babies born at low birthweights does not mean that prenatal care is useless or ineffective. During these same years, infant mortality continued to drop. The expansions of Medicaid were quite effective in improving the health of children. But they did not achieve that goal, it seems, by preventing low birthweight and thus decreasing the need for neonatal intensive care. Instead, they seemed to work by more comprehensively identifying the highest-risk mothers, transferring them to tertiary care centers, and ensuring that they received the best obstetric and neonatal care available. Prenatal care, far from decreasing the need for intensive care, seemed to increase it.

These facts put to rest the apparent controversy about whether we spend too much on neonatal interventions and not enough on prevention. These two approaches to infant mortality are not, in reality, an either-or choice. They appear to be so only when they are opposed to each other for political purposes. Clearly, the best thing for babies is not to choose between one and the other, but to build systems that seamlessly provide both. Such systems do not reduce costs, but they do improve outcomes.

Discarded moral view 2: Neonatology should be curtailed because the harms caused by the increased numbers of survivors with cerebral palsy and other neurological deficits outweigh the benefits of increased survival rates.

In 1992, Paneth wrote, "Surely it is now time for national organizations of neonatologists to gather together and set a threshold of birth weight and gestational age below which ordinarily (there may be individual exceptions) it is inadvisable to apply the technology of newborn intensive care."[11] The next year, Hack and Fanaroff suggested that the care of extremely premature babies was experimental because the true long-term harms had not been assessed. As an experimental treatment, they suggested, it should be carefully monitored and perhaps curtailed.[12] Around the same time, Oregon developed a rationing plan that, had it been implemented, would not have paid for neonatal intensive care for babies below 500 grams birthweight.[13] In a commentary, Silverman suggested that the treatment of these babies had more to do with the grandiosity of the doctors than the interests of either the babies or their parents.[14]

This moral critique of neonatology was not directed at the entire field but at the treatment at the very margins, the treatment of the babies at the lowest birthweights and thus at the highest risk for bad outcomes. In essence, this was an argument about the quality of life for survivors and the costs associated with survival with a quality of life that was perceived to be poor and thus not worth the expenditures. By this argument, the partial successes of neonatology in the treatment of these high-risk babies was outweighed by the social, economic, and emotional costs of the partial failures. On an individual level, such considerations lead to the sorts of considerations that are the focus of clinical ethics and might lead to decisions, in individual cases, to discontinue life-sustaining treatment. On the societal level, they lead to arguments for curtailing treatment for entire classes of babies, usually defined by birthweight or gestational age.

These societal-level arguments turn, then, on the effect that neonatal intensive care has had on society as a whole. The key question is whether, as a result of neonatal intensive care, the overall burden of lifelong neurological deficits has increased. In other words, is neonatology making our society less healthy instead of more healthy?

Interestingly, it has been difficult to determine the effect that neonatal intensive care has had on the overall rates of cerebral palsy (CP) or other neurological conditions. As with the controversy about prenatal care as a means to prevent low birthweight, this one turns, at least partially, on the facts. If the prevalence of cerebral palsy is, in fact, increasing, and if that can, in fact, be attributed to the NICU, then the argument against NICU care for the highest-risk babies has more resonance than if that is not the case. The debate about whether this is true has been heated, methodologically complex, and inconclusive.

The debate begins with the uncontroversial recognition that many extremely premature babies who survive are left with neurodevelopmental problems. This was true in the earliest days of neonatology and remains true today, as shown by two recent studies looking at long-term outcomes for extremely low-birthweight babies. Anderson and Doyle studied nearly 300 babies born in the early 1990s whose birthweight was less than 1000 grams and compared them with normal birthweight controls. They found that "school-age children born ELBW or very preterm in the 1990s continue to display more cognitive, educational, and behavioral impairments relative to NBW controls. More than 50 percent of ELBW or very preterm children exhibited a clinically significant impairment."[15] Similarly, Saigal and colleagues studied more than 500 babies from four countries who weighed between 500 and 1000 grams at birth. They found, "The proportion of children who performed within the normal range (> or =85) were as follows: IQ between 44% and 62%; reading between 46% and 81%; arithmetic between 31% and 76%; and spelling between 39% and 65% . . . More than half of all cohorts required special educational assistance and/or repeated a grade."[16]

These data raise two questions: First, are these sorts of long-term outcomes so bad that death would be preferable? This question can be answered only by the developing ways of assessing quality of life and using those assessments to decide which babies might be allowed to die. We have already discussed the complexities of such assessments. The second question raised by these data is whether the high incidence of CP among the tiniest babies is leads to an increased prevalence of CP in the population of children as a whole. Are the problems in the smallest babies outweighed by improvements among larger babies? In other words, is the overall prevalence of CP rising, staying the same, or decreasing as a result of neonatal interventions? It seems plausible to suggest that it is rising, because there are so many more survivors of neonatal intensive care overall. However, perhaps improvements in obstetric care and in the care of larger babies lead to an overall decrease in cerebral palsy that offsets modest rises in the rate of CP in the lower birthweight groups.

Different studies suggest conflicting answers to these questions. Wichers and colleagues studied CP rates in the Netherlands.[17] They concluded, "CP prevalence rose significantly over time: from 0.77 (1977–1979) to 2.44 (1986–1988)." They did not examine the relative contribution of low birthweight or prematurity.

Pharoah and colleagues in Liverpool created a register of all cases of cerebral palsy in two counties in England over the past three decades. They claim, "The prevalence of cerebral palsy has increased among all the low birthweight groups with, most recently, an increase in infants weighing <1000 g at birth. Low birthweight infants now comprise about 50% of all cases of cerebral palsy; in the early years of the study they comprised about 32% of all cases."[18] Although their data suggest that the proportion of CP cases attributable to low birthweight has steadily risen over the years, they do not see the same magnitude of overall increase that was seen by Wichers and colleagues.

Clark recently reviewed a number of studies from a several countries and concluded that the overall rates of CP are staying about the same. Furthermore, rates seem to be the same in different parts of the world, even parts of the world with vastly different usages of neonatal intensive care. For example, the prevalence of CP in China, India, and Slovenia is similar to that in the United States, England, and Canada.[19]

Lorenz and colleagues did a systematic literature review of forty-two studies published since 1970. They found that, "the prevalence of disabilities had not changed . . . with increasing survival. However, increasing survival of these (premature) infants has resulted in a steadily increasing prevalence of children with disabilities."[20] Winter and colleagues find a similar stability in the prevalence of CP among low-birthweight survivors between 1975 and 1991. Contributing to these surprising findings is the increased prevalence of CP among normal birthweight babies.[21]

Part of the reason for the conflicting results and the inconclusiveness of the data relate to the complexity of the problems being studied. Nobody knows what causes CP. Some cases seem to be clearly related to perinatal or neonatal events, but the majority of cases have no apparent cause. Furthermore, the effects of NICU care cannot be analyzed in isolation. During the era in question, there were many changes in obstetric care, in the organization of perinatal services, in the use of in vitro fertilization, and in the follow-up care of high-risk newborns. Many premature babies are followed in NICU follow-up clinics. As a result, it may be easier to ascertain subtle cases of CP among those babies than among full-term babies. In addition, cerebral palsy itself is a diagnosis that presents with a wide spectrum of physical and cognitive findings. Thus, it is not a straightforward diagnosis to make.

Despite these somewhat conflicting results and the methodologic problems, some tentative conclusions can be drawn. Neonatology does appear not to lead to or cause an increased overall societal prevalence of cerebral palsy. Instead, neonatology has shifted the patterns of causation of cerebral palsy. The lowest birthweight survivors of neonatal intensive care clearly are at high risk for such CP. Slightly larger babies are, today, at lower risk than they were. The critique of neonatology based on the fear that it was imposing a large new burden on society by creating more severely disabled survivors is not borne out by the facts. Instead, the picture that emerges from these studies is more morally complicated. A greater proportion of cerebral palsy today may be attributable to decisions that we make about treatment or nontreatment of babies than was the case in the part.

One way to think about this is to imagine that, in the past, cerebral palsy occurred in ways over which we had no control. Now, we are responsible in a whole new way. This recognition focuses concern less on the overall cost-benefit or cost-effectiveness analyses and more on the attitudes of doctors, parents, and society in general toward people with disabilities.

Discarded moral view 3: Parents alone should have the final say as to whether their babies are treated.

From the earliest days of neonatology, there was concern that many parents did not want their babies to be saved, especially if the babies would be left with neurological deficits. This concern was the focus of the articles by Duff and Campbell and by Shaw in the early 1970s that began the public debate about neonatal ethics. It was incorporated into the recommendations of the President's Commission on Bioethics in 1982. Those recommendations stated that, in circumstances where the outcome of treatment would be "ambiguous or uncertain," the parents' opinions should determine treatment. American common law enshrines the right of competent adults to privacy and autonomy in making medical decisions and extends that right to children through their parents. All of these authoritative sources lend credence to the idea that parents should be permitted to reject treatment for a newborn baby in any circumstance in which they could reject treatment for themselves.

Two of the most eloquent proponents of this view, over the years, have been neonatologist William Silverman and Jesuit priest John Paris. Silverman was one of the pioneers of neonatology and has become one of its strongest critics. He argues that many of the efforts of neonatologists lead to outcomes that destroy the lives of parents and families. He writes,

> Parents, struggling to rear severely retarded children born after extreme prematurity, protest that they were "made to feel like criminals for questioning" heroic medical treatment. Doctors are "out of touch with the harsh realities of our children's

lives," they complain. "Where," they ask, "is a description of the months or years of grueling hospitalization with the associated gastrostomy tubes, jejunostomy tubes, and fundoplications; the tracheostomies, shunts, orthopedic, eye, and brain surgeries; hyperalimentation, oxygen tanks, and ventilators?" Similarly, medical accounting fails to recognize the frequency of emotional and financial breakdown in families caused by the extreme burdens of caring for developmentally retarded children with super-imposed severe medical problems.[22]

John Paris, in a critical analysis of the case of *Miller v. HCA*, notes, "respect for individual choice has, till now, been applied to treatment decisions made by parents for infants born at the margin of viability."[23] He cites the 1995 joint report of the American Academy of Pediatrics Committee on Fetus and Newborns and American College of Obstetrics and Gynecologists Committee on Obstetric Practice which states that, "Decisions regarding obstetric management must be made by the parents and their physicians if the neonate's prognosis is uncertain."[24] The report notes that counseling on the available data on the child's status "may result in the family choosing a noninterventive approach to delivery and management." Paris concludes that "the expectation is that it is both legitimate and anticipated that parents, once informed of the risks of marked prematurity, are the ones to make the decision on whether or not to utilize aggressive interventions or to provide 'comfort care' for their child."

Despite these official endorsements and eloquent defenses of parents' rights, there are two problems with this approach to decision making. The first is that the assertion that parents have the right to make treatment decisions with regard to their children ignores the child's independent moral status and sometimes conflicting right to potentially beneficial medical treatment. Given this right, the scope of parental discretion is necessarily limited to the freedom to make only those decisions that are in the child's interests. This, of course, begs the question of whether parents are better at making that determination than doctors, judges, or legislators.

A second problem with this approach is its implicit assumption that, in general, parents are less likely to desire treatment than doctors will be to recommend it. In most cases, the opposite is true—parents are, in general, much more likely to want treatment that doctors think is futile than they are to refuse treatment that doctors think is efficacious. As a result, the procedural formula for decision making that uniquely empowers parents often leads to situations in which parents demand treatment that is expensive and ineffective. In those situations, ironically, some philosophers who argue for parents' rights when the parents are choosing nontreatment argue against parental discretion. Paris, for example, suggests that, when doctors think treatment is futile, parents should not have the right to insist that it continue.[25]

Neither doctors nor parents are always right or always should have the right to make decisions. Instead, the best decisions often result from a collective decision-making process in which parents, other family members, doctors, nurses, and ethicists collaborate to try to understand what choices best reflect the interests of the babies. Neither doctors nor parents are unconstrained in the way that they used to be. Both are subject to judicial scrutiny and both are held to publicly articulated standards for decision making. Debate now turns on specific facts and circumstances of particular cases and the careful weighing of the child's interests against the parents' rights.

Discarded moral view 4: Respect for the sanctity of life demands that we never consider "quality of life" in deciding whether to discontinue life-sustaining treatment.

The term "quality of life" has multiple meanings. In some contexts, it is used to refer to the subjective assessments of competent adults as to their own sense of happiness or well being. As such, it is an important complement to objective measures of outcome. In other contexts, such as the one in which decisions must be made about treatment of critically ill newborns, the term refers to a third party's assessment of the suffering or the burdens experienced by a patient who is unable to express his or her own opinions. In that context, in particular, quality-of-life assessments have been particularly problematic. Part of the rationale for curtailing parental discretion was a belief that each baby's life was sacred. Some extended this argument to suggest that medical treatment could never be withheld or withdrawn without starting a long slide toward Nazi-era policies of trying to eliminate all citizens with disabilities of any sort.

Pediatric surgeon C. Everett Koop made this argument in 1977, "We are rapidly moving from the state of mind where destruction of life is advocated for children who are considered to be socially useless or have non-meaningful lives to a place where we are willing to destroy a child because he is socially disturbing. What we need is alternatives, either in the form of education or palliative measures for the individual as well as for society. We here should be old enough to know that history does teach lessons. Destructiveness eventually is turned on the destroyer and self-destruction is the result. If you do not believe me, look at Nazi Germany."[26] By the 1980s, Koop was surgeon general of the United States and tried to incorporate these concerns and fears into the federal regulations governing treatment decisions in the NICU.

His efforts to do so, paradoxically, made clear the inevitability of incorporating some consideration of quality of life into decision making. The alternative, it seemed, was not heightened moral sensibility but a morally insensitive zealotry that would have enslaved babies to a vitalist ideology. If quality of life was not considered in any way, then it would be necessary to continue treatment of all babies with every available technology until the last heartbeat. Theologian Richard McCormick summarized the problems we would thus encounter, "The availability of powerful new technologies that can sustain life almost indefinitely has forced us to ask: what are we doing when we intervene to stave off death? What values are we seeking to serve? How should we formulate these values in our time if we are to maintain (individually and collectively) our grasp on the basic values that define our well-being? Ought we sustain life when the individual gains nothing from such sustenance? And what does 'stand to gain nothing' mean?"[27]

Clearly, we have discarded a number of moral views in coming to the current tentative consensus. We have replaced them with a set of principles and practices that are tentative, imperfect, and the result of compromises between various factions and moral impulses. As a society, we have made a serious commitment to both prenatal and neonatal intensive care. As a society, we have shown a willingness to prohibit some quality-of-life decisions but to allow others. As a society, we have decided that neither doctors nor parents alone may decide when life-sustaining treatment ought to be withheld or withdrawn. Instead, doctors and parents together must agree to stop treatment or else treatment will continue. This approach is expensive but it saves lives, preserves important moral values, and does not seem to have morally intolerable long-term sequelae for individuals, families, or society. We continue to evaluate and scrutinize these practices and to make adjustments in the prevailing consensus as new information becomes available. The prevailing morality is thus as open ended as the prevailing science and technology. It is a consensus in which we must have the courage to allow ourselves doubt.

CHAPTER EIGHT

The Possibility of Moral Progress

A cartoon compares science and ethics. In the top half, there is a picture of a quadruped, walking across the frame from left to right. In each successive frame, the creature evolves. He begins as a small ape, becomes half-human, then a primitive human, and finally a civilized, well-dressed modern man. This part of the cartoon is labeled "Science." The bottom half of the cartoon shows the same quadruped on the left, but as he walks across the frame, he does not evolve. He looks exactly the same on the right side of the cartoon as he did on the left. This part of the cartoon is labeled "Ethics."

The cartoon implies that science has made enormous progress over the years but that ethics has not and never will. The cartoon picks up on a familiar intuition that ethical problems are irresolvable, that ethical arguments are inherently, inevitably, and irreducibly circular. It sometimes seems that way; we discuss the problems endlessly but never end up with any more certainty about the right thing to do than we had when we started. This is reflected in the timelessness of ethics expertise. After all, in ethics, we still read the ancient masters along with more modern philosophers. All are still relevant. In the sciences, by contrast, only the latest writings are relevant. The knowledge is cumulative. New discoveries replace and invalidate previously held beliefs. We move forward, ever increasing our knowledge, getting closer and closer to complex truths about the way the world is. The science of the ancient masters is only of historical interest. If they were wrong, it is quaint. If they were right, their work has been incorporated into newer paradigms.

This view of the contrast between science and ethics is true in one sense but misleading in another. The task, in ethics, is not to discover new truths but instead to figure out how to apply ancient principles to new problems. Furthermore, the goal of ethics is not to progress beyond ancient wisdom but instead to help each person relearn the truths in ways that enable them to incorporate those truths into their lives. Each person, as they move through their lives, will face dilemmas about how to be moral. Each will face situations where he or she will have to decide what it means to be fair, loyal, honest, courageous, or loving. Each of us comes to some individual understanding of the world and our place in it. In reaching such understandings, ancient wisdom is still relevant because the basic elements of human relationships and human choices have not changed over time. And new analyses of ancient truths are equally relevant; the precise nature of the choices we face and the dilemmas we must address are new, different, and complex. We have always worried about death and dying, but the circumstances surrounding those events admit new choices today.

This understanding of the important ways in which ethical knowledge can be both timeless and of-the-moment is true in a universal way for every human being as they move through life. It is also true in a particular way for different individuals in specific circumstances. So, in medicine, for example, each doctor has to learn the norms and values of the profession and make choices about the particular behaviors that will uphold those norms. Some of the dilemmas and some of the choices are unchanged since Hippocrates. Doctors, uniquely, have always had to decide whether to tell their patients the truth, whether to protect confidentiality, and how to handle situations such as sexual attraction for a patient. The dilemmas are always slightly different in their particulars but always fundamentally the same in their themes. Each individual has to struggle with the issues that every other individual has always struggled with.

It is misleading, however, to suggest that, because the dilemmas are timeless and eternal, and because each individual must relearn ancient wisdom for himself or herself, that therefore we do not make progress. The relevant contrast is not between scientific progress and moral stasis. Instead, it is between science and art as two different ways of interrogating the world and ourselves. Learning to be a moral person is more like learning to be a piano player or a potter than it is like conducting an experiment. To learn how to play the newest tunes, we must learn to play the oldest. In every age, we aspire to an ancient and timeless ideal. An excellent piano player today does not have to be "better" or to "know more" than his or her counterpart of 100 or 200 years ago. Today's ceramics are not "better" than those of the Han dynasty. Instead, the goal is to master the timeless techniques of a craft and then to use those techniques to inform life and work. Similarly, the goal in ethics is to understand the wisdom of the ages and to apply it to the circumstances of the present. This task is neither circular nor static. It is dynamic and creative.

Within this broad task, then, we can think of progress differently than we think about scientific progress. New discoveries, new technologies, and new cultural arrangements lead to new moral dilemmas. To come up with solutions, these dilemmas first have to be analyzed and characterized. We need to understand just how they are similar to and how they are different from problems that have come before. We need to figure out how to apply the timeless norms and values that should never be compromised. These tasks lead us to new understandings of ourselves, our place in the world, and what life is all about.

The dilemmas surrounding neonatal intensive care are a particularly rich example of such a process. Scientific discoveries and technological inventions enabled us, for the first time in human history, to save the lives of critically ill newborns. These same discoveries forced us to reexamine what it means to be a parent, or a doctor, or a just society. We had to rethink the value of human life at the very extreme of life. Premature babies, born months too soon, or babies with complex congenital anomalies, have seemed throughout human history to be barely human. In many societies and in many historical eras, they were not given the same moral status or rights as older persons. Their extreme vulnerability is such that their very survival would depend not just on tolerance or acceptance but instead on the creation of a complex organization of human and economic and social capital. As this field was being invented, it was not clear whether such efforts were a good thing or a bad thing, whether they would lead to more harms or benefits, whether they were worth the enormous investment that they would demand.

A steady increase in the clinical efficacy of these therapies gradually created tenuous and contested new facts. The process of fact creation was itself the subject of ethical reflection. Clinical research on neonates required an examination of the moral norms that governed medical innovation-patient selection, study design, informed consent, and the appropriate distribution of the risks and benefits of research. New solutions were proposed, some were adopted, some discarded. The issue is still very controversial. But the tentative compromises allowed data to be collected and analyzed in a way that formed the substrate for a new set of ethical conundrums that followed. As doctors incorporated new discoveries into routine clinical practice, they were able to save tinier and sicker babies than they had ever been able to save before. Nobody knew the risk-benefit ratios of these treatments in different circumstances. Would they work for babies under 3 pounds, or 2, or 1?

Did they have unforeseen side effects? Would the babies whose lives were saved be left with chronic problems, such as blindness or seizures or cerebral palsy? And if lives could be saved but only with residual disabilities, was that a net benefit or a net harm? And who should decide?

The forward movement of neonatal bioethics occurred as these questions were transformed from theoretical speculations to practical dilemmas in the lives of doctors, nurses, judges, and parents. As that happened, the ethical issues shifted from topics for speculation about whether hypothetical treatments of imaginary babies might or might not be morally obligatory. Instead, the questions became grounded in the particular circumstances of a particular family facing a particular decision at a particular time and in a particular place. At that point, all of the theoretical responses collapsed like a wave function in particle physics. The urgent need was no longer for elegant arguments. It was for a particular answer about a particular baby. Should we intubate this baby, now, in the delivery room of this hospital? If we do not, the baby will surely die. If we do, we step into the unknown. The baby might die a more prolonged and painful death. The baby might be saved by a few days of judicious medical treatment. The baby might survive with horrendous brain damage.

Once the technology became available, a decision could no longer be avoided. Technology does not create a moral imperative for its own use. We can, after all, decide not to use it. But technology does create a moral imperative to choose, to decide whether and how to use it. There is no longer an option to not choose. The imperative to make a choice devolves on the individuals involved in each particular case.

A further imperative is also created—the imperative to understand the basis for the decision and to create societal mechanisms for allowing preferential decisions to be made. A proper response to this aspect of the moral imperative of technology requires input from epidemiology, physiology, law, philosophy, economics, psychology, theology, public policy, gender studies, literature, and many other areas of inquiry. The difficulty is that conversations across such disparate disciplines are often garbled in translation. One of the roles of modern bioethics is to straddle the boundaries, to facilitate meaningful dialogue between the doctors, lawyers, philosophers, theologians, economists, and social scientists whose inquiries are all important to our coming up with the best moral response.

This book argues for a particular type of moral progress. We use neonatal intensive care as an example of the complex interplay of scientific discovery, technological innovation, moral searching, legal oversight, regulatory superstructures, and philosophical explorations. Together, these efforts led to a societal consensus about how to take care of the most vulnerable of our citizens. In each of these zones of discourse and discovery, dilemmas that once seemed puzzling or insoluble have been dealt with productively. We have figured out how to harness ambiguous technology to human ends.

Medicine has clearly become too important a societal matter to be left to either physicians or medical administrators. It has become the central political project of modern industrial societies. The United States has a free-market economy and a democratic political system, both of which are designed to ensure that the allocation of resources is driven by the preferences and choices of individual consumers or voters. Under that citizen-driven system, we devote 16 percent of our enormous economic resources to health care. We decide, collectively, to spend nearly $2 trillion every year on health. We are all inevitably concerned about and involved with decisions about how that money is or ought to be spent. The task of evaluating new medical projects and deciding whether they are wise, desirable, or worthy engages all of us. The more subtle task of deciding the limits of medical projects and specifying the proper locus of control for decisions to delimit the scope of medical interventions is also, necessarily, a public and therefore political responsibility.

In the early twenty-first century, our university, like so many others around the world, is in the process of dramatically expanding its commitment to both biomedical research and to clinical medicine. We have opened a stunning new children's hospital that will have many more NICU beds than our current children's hospital. We are building many new research laboratories. One of our new buildings will be devoted to collaborations between physicists and biologists who together will try to understand the fundamental nature of physical and chemical reactions within cells. A new Institute for Molecular Pediatrics will try to nudge the field of pediatrics toward a deeper and more refined understanding of the fundamental mechanisms of health and disease in childhood. A new Center for Health and the Social Sciences will bring together biological scientists, sociologists, and economists who will try to understand how to best focus our material and intellectual resources to improve people's health. Our Center for Clinical Medical Ethics is a flourishing multidisciplinary enterprise that fosters collaboration between clinicians, scientists, and scholars in the humanities to analyze and understand the implications of our new knowledge and new technology.

The medical care of the premature and critically ill newborns who are admitted to our new NICU will be financed collectively through either taxpayer dollars or through the virtually mandatory contributions that most of us make to employer-sponsored (and tax-sheltered) health care plans. The research that will take place in our new research laboratories and centers will be financed through taxpayer dollars that flow through the National Institutes of Health and by generous private donations. The hospital and the university are private, not-for-profit institutions, governed by community boards, and dependent on the financial contributions of members of the community. Clearly, this work could not go forward without massive collective public and private support. It relies on a public mandate.

Clearly, too, the mechanisms for governance of this multidisciplinary enterprise are not straightforward. There is no health care czar, no single entity that makes the hard decisions, no single newspaper or journal that we can turn to, to understand what decisions are coming up for a vote. Instead, there is only the collective pushing and pulling of multiple interest groups, hundreds of lobbies, thousands of micromarkets, and millions of people with needs or desires of one sort or another.

The goings-on in the new and improved NICU in our new children's hospital and in other NICUs throughout the country will roughly conform to the values that have been described in this book. Collectively, though not formally, we have made rules that govern the practices of the doctors, nurses, and parents who together must make choices regarding the babies. One of the joys and burdens of living in a secular, pluralist democratic society is that we must make our own rules. We decide what values we want to uphold, what institutions we want to support, what sorts of relationships and obligations we want to prioritize. And we decide which sorts of values, institutions, and relationships we want to forbid. We may say, for example, that physician-assisted suicide, gay marriage, or abortion are legal or illegal. We may allow parents to refuse treatment for a baby with Down syndrome, or not. We may direct funding toward the NICU, toward the primary care clinic, or toward injury-prevention programs. We may vote to expand Medicaid programs or to cut their budgets.

The answers that we have come to about decisions in the NICU were not in any way obvious at the start. They are not settled or final. The process of arriving at moral consensus is iterative, nonlinear, and ongoing. Scientific discoveries challenge us to change the way we think about the potential for particular projects. These projects may, in turn, change the way we think about what it means to be human and what it means to live in community. Things that once seemed good may, over time, seem problematic. We change the way we view cars, or pesticides, or nuclear fission, or life-sustaining medical technology. Usually, we do not accept or reject an innovation outright. We modify it. We regulate it. We build on the initial discoveries to develop new and perhaps safer ways of deploying the new innovations. Sometimes, new possibilities for human flourishing emerge. But each new possibility is as double-stranded as a DNA molecule, holding within it both hopes and fears, risks and benefits, dangers and possibilities for the escape from danger. Each story of scientific discovery and innovation is a story of the struggle to find the balance between the two.

Once we know what we *can* do, we begin to ask whether we *should*. Competing ideas about the human good are proposed. There is, perhaps, one fundamental question at the center of all bioethical debate: "Is it worth it?" We take it for granted that it is our task to improve the human condition. We debate whether any particular effort in that direction is likely to succeed and, if so, if it is the best way to expend our financial and moral and psychological and intellectual resources to shape our lives and our communities around a particular vision of the good. This is a particularly vexing task in a society like ours because such societies have no universally held vision of the good. Instead, visions of the good compete with one another and are forever conditional, evolving, negotiable.

It sometimes seems unclear whether our health care system as a whole and the biomedical research enterprise as a whole are on the right track. The transition of scientific discoveries from the laboratory bench to a patient's bedside, from interesting conceptual breakthrough to practical application, is often long and complex. The story of neonatology is an interesting paradigm case of one such journey. In the last leg of such journeys from bench to bedside, questions of ethics and human values come to the fore in new and compelling ways.

The story of neonatology suggests that, although our ideas of what is good or right do not flow straightforwardly from traditional sources, they nevertheless are ideas that we can articulate, clarify, and then impose on ourselves. The story is about the process by which we tack back and forth between different and often opposing moral views, eventually finding a course to take that allows tentative collective action. At each stage, we make a tentative collective choice to accept a certain morality. We observe the effects. We move forward. We change.

Some are frightened by this sort of approach to morality and imagine that we should be more certain of moral solutions than we are of scientific solutions. Such fears have, for example, led some to call for a moratorium on certain forms of biomedical research until we can better understand the moral implications. Thus, the President's Council on Bioethics has written,

> We believe that a permanent ban on cloning-to-produce-children coupled with a four-year moratorium on cloning-for-biomedical-research would be the best way for our society to express its firm position on the former, and to engage in a properly informed and open democratic deliberation on the latter . . . The decision before us is of great moment and importance. Creating cloned embryos for any purpose requires crossing a major moral boundary, with grave risks and likely harms, and once we

cross it there will be no turning back. Our society should take the time to do it right and to make a judgment that is well informed and morally sound, respectful of strongly held views, and representative of the priorities and principles of the American people." The mechanism that the President's Council endorses is a legislative ban on such research until society has had the time to way the risks and benefits.[1]

Societal oversight of the biomedical research enterprise is entirely appropriate. Committees review every project that involves research on human subjects to ensure that it is scientifically sound, that subjects are informed of the risks and benefits, that they freely consent to participation, and that they may withdraw from projects at any time. Not every project that is imagined by scientists should be endorsed by society. Some projects are so morally problematic at the outset that they should be prohibited. It is both proper and necessary to analyze the trade-offs between the risks of innovation and the risks of doing nothing.

However, it is impossible to quantify, weigh, and measure the risks and benefits without first trying to do things and seeing if they work. In searching for answers, we began to understand the questions. Each solution leads to new hypotheses. We could learn only by doing, and, in doing, we learn what we need to explore next. The disorderly and unpredictable process continues. Because scientific discoveries carry within them the seeds of both triumph and tragedy, we need to be attentive and cautious to the possibilities that our deepest hopes might lead us to create our worst nightmares.

The paradigm of neonatology as a success story of modern medicine and modern bioethics has implications for other areas of biomedical innovation. The fundamental clash, at the outset, was between a moral stance by which each baby was seen as an independent moral agent with rights that needed to be recognized and protected, or whether, instead, each baby was seen as a potential moral agent whose survival depended primarily on his or her parents' choices. The moral decision to invest each baby with moral worth and corresponding moral rights was a radical departure from the past. Each of the dilemmas that followed—whether a baby with Down syndrome must be treated, whether to try to save babies whose prognosis is uncertain, when and whether to deem treatments futile, how to conduct clinical research—became an effort to apply the moral principle to the particular circumstances.

The ethics of biomedical innovation will get more and more complicated as knowledge and power increase. Hope must be tempered with humility and fear with courage if we are to find the balance that we need to harness amoral technology to human ends.

Notes

CHAPTER 1: OVERVIEW AND INTRODUCTION

1. Preemies: Baby Doe law creates miracles—at a cost. *San Luis Obispo County Telegram Tribune*. March 9, 1998.

2. Paris JJ, and Reardon F. Bad cases make bad law: *HCA v. Miller* is not a guide for resuscitation of extremely premature newborns. *J Perinatol* 2001;21:541–44.

3. Annas GJ. Extremely preterm birth and parental authority to refuse treatment: the case of Sidney Miller. *N Engl J Med* 2004;351:2118–23.

4. Whittier G. The ethics of metaphor and the infant body in pain. *Literature and Medicine* 1999;18:210–35.

5. Wichers MJ, van der Schouw YT, Moons KG, Stam HJ, and van Nieuwenhuizen O. Prevalence of cerebral palsy in The Netherlands (1977–1988). *Eur J Epidemiol* 2001;17(6): 7–32.

6. Winter S, Autry A, Boyle C, and Yeargin-Allsopp M. Trends in the prevalence of cerebral palsy in a population-based study. *Pediatrics* December 2002;110(6):1220–25.

7. Anspach R. *Deciding Who Lives: Fateful Choices in the Intensive Care Nursery.* Berkeley: U. of California, 1997.

CHAPTER 2: SOME FACTS ABOUT INFANT MORTALITY AND NEONATAL CARE

1. Lee KS, Khoshnood B, Hsieh H, Kim BI, Schreiber MD, and Mittendorf R. Which infant groups contributed most to the overall reduction in the neonatal mortality rates in the United States from 1960 to 1986? *Paediatr Perinat Epidemiol* 1995;9:420–30.

CHAPTER 3: THE ERA OF INNOVATION AND INDIVIDUALISM, 1965–1982

1. Florey HW. Penicillin. Nobel lecture, December 11, 1945. Available at: http://nobelprize.org/medicine/laureates/1945/florey-lecture.pdf. Accessed November 9, 2005.

2. Mailer JS, and Mason B. Penicillin: medicine's wartime wonder drug and its production at Peoria, Illinois. Available at: www.lib.niu.edu/ipo/iht810139.html. Accessed November 9, 2005.

3. Osler W. *The Principles and Practice of Medicine.* New York: D Appleton & Co., 1898: 109–12.

4. Johnson AH, Peacock JL, Greenough A, Marlow N, Limb ES, Marston L, Calvert SA, and United Kingdom Oscillation Study Group. High-frequency oscillatory ventilation for the prevention of chronic lung disease of prematurity. *N Engl J Med* 2002;347:633–42.

5. Silverman WA. A cautionary tale about supplemental oxygen: the albatross of neonatal medicine. *Pediatrics* 2004;113:394–96.

6. Delivoria-Papadopoulos M, Levinson H, and Swyer PR. Intermittent positive pressure respiration as a treatment in severe respiratory distress syndrome. *Arch Dis Child* 1965;40:474–79.

7. Dr. Maria Delavoria-Papadopoulos, personal communication, May 3, 2004.

8. Delivoria-Papadopoulos et al., *Arch Dis Child* 40:475.

9. Ibid., 476.

10. Ibid., 479.

11. Cooke R, Friis-Hansen B, and Lunding M. Endotracheal tube fixation and postural drainage in prolonged artificial ventilation of the newborn: description of a new apparatus. *Acta Paediatr Scand* 1967;56:509–12.

12. Reid DH, and Tunstall ME. Treatment of respiratory-distress syndrome of newborn with nasotracheal intubation and intermittent positive-pressure respiration. *Lancet* June 1965;33:1196–97.

13. Tunstall ME, Cater JI, Thomson JS, and Mitchell RG. Ventilating the lungs of newborn infants for prolonged periods. *Arch Dis Child* 1968 43:486–97.

14. Gregory GA, Kitterman JA, Phibbs RH, Tooley WH, and Hamilton WK. Treatment of the idiopathic respiratory-distress syndrome with continuous positive airway pressure. *N Engl J Med* 1971;284:1333–40.

15. Ibid.

16. Ibid.

17. Ibid., 1338.

18. Chernick V. Continuous distending pressure in hyaline membrane disease: of devices, disadvantages, and a daring study. *Pediatrics* 1973;52(1):114–15.

19. Dudrick SJ. Early developments and clinical applications of total parenteral nutrition. *J Parenter Enteral Nutr* 2003;27:291–99.

20. Ibid., 294.

21. Wilmore DW, Groff DB, Bishop HC, and Dudrick SJ. Total parenteral nutrition in infants with catastrophic gastrointestinal anomalies. *J Pediatr Surg* 1969;4:181–89.

22. Winters RW. Total parenteral nutrition in pediatrics: the Borden award address. *Pediatrics* 1975 Jul;56(1):17–23.

23. Chernick, *Pediatrics.*

24. Lucey JF, ed., Problems of neonatal intensive care units. 59th Ross Conference on Pediatric Research; Ross Laboratories; Columbus, Ohio; 1968.

25. Ibid.

26. Moore TD, ed. Ethical dilemmas in current obstetrics and newborn care. 65th Ross Conference; Ross Laboratories; Columbus, Ohio; 1972.

27. Ibid.

28. Ibid.

29. Jonsen AR, Phibbs RH, Tooley WH, and Garland MJ. Critical issues in newborn intensive care: a conference report and policy proposal. *Pediatrics* 1975;55:756–65.

30. Swyer PR. The regional organization of special care for the neonate. *Pediatr Clin North Am* 1970;17:761–76.

31. Finkler SA. Cost-effectiveness of regionalization: the heart surgery example. *Inquiry* Fall 1979;16(3):264–70.

32. Peterson OL, and Bloom BS. Regionalization of surgical services. *Am J Public Health* 1983;73(2):179–83.

33. Luft HS. Regionalization of medical care. *Am J Public Health* 1985;75(2):125–26.

34. Butterfield LJ. The impact of regionalization on neonatal outcomes. In Smith GF, and Vidyasaggar D, eds. *Historic Review and Recent Advances in Neonatal and Perinatal Medicine.* Mead Johnson, 1980. Available at: www. neonatology.org/ classics/ mj1980/ ch22.html. Accessed October 2005.

35. Ryan GM, Pettigrew AH, Fogerty S, and Donahue CL. Regionalizing perinatal health services in Massachusetts. *N Engl J Med* 1977;296:228–30.

36. Sunshine P, ed., Regionalization of perinatal care. 65th Ross Conference on Pediatric Research; Ross Laboratories; Columbus, Ohio; 1974.

37. Ibid.

38. Gould JB, Sarnoff R, Liu H, Bell DR, and Chavez G. Very low birth weight births at non-NICU hospitals: the role of sociodemographic, perinatal, and geographic factors. *J Perinatol* April–May 1999;19(3):197–205.

39. Mehta S, Atherton HD, Schoettker PJ, Hornung RW, Perlstein PH, and Kotagal UR. Differential markers for regionalization. *J Perinatol* September 2000;20(6):366–72.

40. Menard MK, Liu Q, Holgren EA, and Sappenfield WM. Neonatal mortality for very low birth weight deliveries in South Carolina by level of hospital perinatal service. *Am J Obstet Gynecol* August 1998;179(2):374–81.

41. Duff RS, and Campbell AG. Moral and ethical dilemmas in the special-care nursery. *N Engl J Med* 1973;289(17):890–94.

42. Ibid.

43. Shaw A. Dilemmas of "informed consent" in children. *N Engl J Med* 1973;289:885–90.

44. Ibid.

45. Gustafson J. Mongolism, parental desires, and the right to life. *Perspect Biol Med* 1973;529–57.

46. Todres ID, Krane D, Howell MC, and Shannon DC. Pediatricians' attitudes affecting decision-making in defective newborns. *Pediatrics* August 1977;60(2):197–201.

47. Robertson JA, and Fost N. Passive euthanasia of defective newborn infants: legal considerations. *J Pediatr* 1976;88:883–89.

48. Ellis TS. Letting defective babies die: who decides. *Am J Law Med* 1982;7:393–423.

49. Child Abuse Prevention and Treatment Act, PL 93-247, 88 Stat 4 (1974).

50. Lund N. Infanticide, physicians, and the law: the "Baby Doe" Amendments to the Child Abuse and Treatment Act. *Am J Law Med* 1984;11:1–29.

51. Rehabilitation Act of 1973, PL 93-112, 87 Stat 355.

52. Ellis JT. Letting defective babies die: who decides? *Am J Law Med* 1982;7:393–423.

53. *Berman v. Allen*, 80 NJ 421, 429, 404 A2d 8, 12 (1979).

54. Maine, Superior Court, Cumberland County. Trial court decision in the Houle Case. *Issues Law Med* 1986;2:237–39.

55. Horwitz ET. Of love and laetrile: medical decision making in a child's best interests. *Am J Law Med* Fall 1979;5(3):271–94.

CHAPTER 4: THE ERA OF EXPOSED IGNORANCE, 1982–1992

1. Chu J, Clements JA, Cotton ER, Klaus MH, Sweet AY, and Tooley WH. Neonatal pulmonary ischemia. Part I: Clinical and physiologic studies. *Pediatrics* 1967;40:709–85.

2. Fujiwara T, Maeta H, Chida S, Morita T, Watabe Y, and Abe T. Artificial surfactant therapy in hyaline membrane disease. *Lancet* 1980;1:55–59.

3. Kwong MS, Egan EA, Notter RH, and Shapiro DL. Double-blind clinical trial of calf lung surfactant extract for the prevention of hyaline membrane disease in extremely premature infants. *Pediatrics* October 1985;76(4):585–92.

4. Raju TN, Vidyasagar D, Bhat R, Sobel D, McCulloch KM, Anderson M, Maeta H, Levy PS, and Furner S. Double-blind controlled trial of single-dose treatment with bovine surfactant in severe hyaline membrane disease. *Lancet* March 1987;1(8534):651–56.

5. Shapiro DL, Notter RH, Morin FC III, Deluga KS, Golub LM, Sinkin RA, Weiss KI, and Cox C. Double-blind, randomized trial of a calf lung surfactant extract administered at birth to very premature infants for prevention of respiratory distress syndrome. *Pediatrics* October 1985;76(4):593–99.

6. Horbar JD, Soll RF, Sutherland JM, Kotagal U, Philip AG, Kessler DL, Little GA, Edwards WH, Vidyasagar D, Raju TN, et al. A multicenter randomized, placebo-controlled trial of surfactant therapy for respiratory distress syndrome. *N Engl J Med* April 1989 13(15); 320:959–65.

7. Fujiwara T, Konishi M, Chida S, Okuyama K, Ogawa Y, Takeuchi Y, Nishida H, Kito H, Fujimura M, Nakamura H, et al. Surfactant replacement therapy with a single postventilatory dose of a reconstituted bovine surfactant in preterm neonates with respiratory distress syndrome: final analysis of a multicenter, double-blind, randomized trial and comparison with similar trials. *Pediatrics* November 1990;86(5):753–64.

8. Bartlett RH, Andrews AF, Toomasian JM, Haiduc NJ, and Gazzaniga AB. Extracorporeal membrane oxygenation for newborn respiratory failure: forty-five cases. *Surgery* 1982;92:425–33.

9. Dworetz AR, Moya FR, Sabo B, Gladstone I, and Gross I. Survival of infants with persistent pulmonary hypertension without extracorporeal membrane oxygenation. *Pediatrics* 1989;84:1–6.

10. O'Rourke PP, Crone RK, Vacanti JP, Ware JH, Lillehei CW, Parad RB, and Epstein MF. Extracorporeal membrane oxygenation and conventional medical therapy in neonates with persistent pulmonary hypertension of the newborn: a prospective randomized study. *Pediatrics* 1989;84:957–63. Bartlett RH, Roloff DW, Cornell RG, Andrews AF, Dillon PW, and Zwischenberger JB. Extracorporeal circulation in neonatal respiratory failure: a prospective randomized study. *Pediatrics* 1985;76:479–87.

11. Roberts TE. Economic evaluation and randomised controlled trial of extracorporeal membrane oxygenation: UK collaborative trial. Extracorporeal Membrane Oxygenation Economics Working Group. *Brit Med J* 1998;317(7163):911–15.

12. Horbar JD, Carpenter J, Buzas J, Soll RF, Suresh G, Bracken MB, Leviton LC, Plsek PE, Sinclair JC, for the members of the Vermont Oxford Network. Timing of initial surfactant treatment for infants 23 to 29 weeks' gestation: is routine practice evidence based? *Pediatrics* 2004;113:1593–1602.

13. Elbourne D, Field D, and Mugford M. Extracorporeal membrane oxygenation for severe respiratory failure in newborn infants. *Cochrane Database Syst Rev* 2002;(1):CD001340.

14. Liggins GC, and Howie RN. A controlled trial of antepartum glucocorticoid treatment for prevention of the respiratory distress syndrome in premature infants. Pediatrics 1972;50:515–25.

15. Caspi E, Schreyer P, Weinraub Z, Reif R, Levi I, and Mundel G. Prevention of the respiratory distress syndrome in premature infants by antepartum glucocorticoid therapy. *Br J Obstet Gynaecol* 1976;83(3):187–93. Block MF, Kling OR, and Crosby WM. Antenatal glucocorticoid therapy for the prevention of respiratory distress syndrome in the premature infant. *Obstet Gynecol* 1977;50(2):186–90. Morrison JC, Whybrew WD, Bucovaz ET, and Schneider JM. Injection of corticosteroids into mother to prevent neonatal respiratory distress syndrome. *Am J Obstet Gynecol* 1978;131(4):358–66. Papageorgiou AN, Desgranges MF, Masson M, Colle E, Shatz R, and Gelfand MM. The antenatal use of betamethasone in the prevention of respiratory distress syndrome: a controlled double-blind study. *Pediatrics* 1979;63(1):73–79. Taeusch HW, Frigoletto F, Kitzmiller J, Avery ME, Hehre A, Fromm B, Lawson E, and Neff RK. Risk of respiratory distress syndrome after prenatal dexamethasone treatment. *Pediatrics* 1979;63(1):64–72. Doran TA, Swyer P, MacMurray B, Mahon W, Enhorning G, Bernstein A, Falk M, and Wood MM. Results of a double-blind controlled study on the use of betamethasone in the prevention of respiratory distress syndrome. *Am J Obstet Gynecol* 1980;136(3):313–20. Teramo K, Hallman M, and Raivio KO. Maternal glucocorticoid in unplanned premature labor: controlled study on the effects of betamethasone phosphate on the phospholipids of the gastric aspirate and on the adrenal cortical function of the newborn infant. *Pediatr Res* 1980;14(4 pt 1):326–29. Effect of antenatal dexamethasone administration on the prevention of respiratory distress syndrome. *Am J Obstet Gynecol* 1981;141(3):276–87. Schmidt PL, Sims ME, Strassner HT, Paul RH, Mueller E, and McCart D. Effect of antepartum glucocorticoid administration upon neonatal respiratory distress syndrome and perinatal infection. *Am J Obstet Gynecol* 1984;148(2):178–86. Iams JD, Talbert ML, Barrows H, and Sachs L. Management of preterm prematurely ruptured membranes: a prospective randomized comparison of observation versus use of steroids and timed delivery. *Am J Obstet Gynecol* 1985;151(1):32–38. Morales WJ, Diebel ND, Lazar AJ, and Zadrozny D. The effect of antenatal dexamethasone administration on the prevention of respiratory distress syndrome in preterm gestations with premature rupture of membranes. *Am J Obstet Gynecol* 1986;154(3):591–95. Gamsu HR, Mulliner BM, Donnai P, and Dash CH. Antenatal administration of betamethasone to prevent respiratory distress syndrome in preterm infants: report of a UK multicentre trial. *Br J Obstet Gynaecol* 1989;96: 401–10.

16. Crowley P, Chalmers I, and Keirse MJ. The effects of corticosteroid administration before preterm delivery: an overview of the evidence from controlled trials. *Br J Obstet Gynaecol* 1990;97(1):11-25.

17. Meadow WL, Bell A, and Sunstein CR. Statistics, not memories: what was the standard of care for administering antenatal steroids to women in preterm labor between 1985 and 2000? *Obstet Gynecol* 2003;102:356-62.

18. National Institutes of Health. Effect of corticosteroids for fetal maturation on perinatal outcome. NIH Consensus Statement. Washington, DC: NIH, 1994;12:1-24.

19. Meadow WL, Bell A, and Sunstein CR. Statistics, not memories: what was the standard of care for administering antenatal steroids to women in preterm labor between 1985 and 2000? *Obstet Gynecol* 2003;102:356-62.

20. Prentice A, and Lind T. Fetal heart rate monitoring during labour: too frequent intervention, too little benefit? *Lancet* 1987;2(8572):1375-77. "Of the eight prospective randomised controlled trials designed to assess its value in obstetric care, four were concerned with mothers defined as being at high-risk, three with normal or low-risk patients, and the eighth with the total population of a maternity hospital over several months. None suggested any major advantage of continuous fetal heart rate monitoring over intermittent surveillance in terms of neonatal mortality, morbidity, cord blood pH values, or the five minute Apgar score. The rates of caesarean section and forceps delivery were higher in the continuously monitored group."

21. Baker CJ, and Edwards MS. Group B streptococcal infections. In: Remington J, and Klein JO, eds. *Infectious Diseases of the Fetus and Newborn Infant*. 4th ed. Philadelphia: WB Saunders Co., 1995:980-1054.

22. American Academy of Pediatrics, Committee on Infectious Diseases and Committee on Fetus and Newborn. Guidelines for prevention of group B streptococcal infection by chemoprophylaxis. *Pediatrics* 1992;90:775-78.

23. Centers for Disease Control and Prevention. Prevention of perinatal group B streptococcal disease: a public health perspective. *MMWR Morb Mortal Wkly Rep* 1996;45(RR-7): 1-24.

24. Yow MD, Mason EO, Leeds LJ, Thompson PK, Clark DJ, and Gardner SE. Ampicillin prevents intrapartum transmission of group B streptococcus. *JAMA* 1979;241:1245-47.

25. Allardice JG, Baskett TF, Seshia MM, Bowman N, and Malazdrewicz R. Perinatal group B streptococcal colonization and infection. *Am J Obstet Gynecol* 1982;142(6 pt 1):617-20. Boyer KM, and Gotoff SP. Prevention of early-onset neonatal group B streptococcal disease with selective intrapartum chemoprophylaxis. *N Engl J Med* 1986;314:1665-69.

26. Velaphi S, Siegel JD, Wendel GD Jr, Cushion N, Eid WM, and Sanchez PJ. Early-onset group B streptococcal infection after a combined maternal and neonatal group B streptococcal chemoprophylaxis strategy. *Pediatrics* 2003;111:541-47.

27. American College of Obstetricians and Gynecologists. Group B streptococcal infections in pregnancy: ACOG's recommendations. *ACOG Newsl* 1993;37:1.

28. Jafari HS, Schuchat A, Hilsdon R, Whitney CG, Toomey KE, and Wenger JD. Barriers to prevention of perinatal group B streptococcal disease. *Pediatr Infect Dis J* 1995;14:662-67.

29. Lukacs SL, Schoendorf KC, and Schuchat A. Trends in sepsis-related neonatal mortality in the United States, 1985-1998. *Pediatr Infect Dis J* 2004;23:599-603.

30. Aoyagi T, Kishi M, Yamaguchi K, and Watanabe S. Improvement of the earpiece oximeter. In: Abstracts of the Japanese Society of Medical Electronics and Biological Engineering, Tokyo 1974:90–91.

31. Barrington KJ, Finer NN, and Ryan CA. Evaluation of pulse oximetry as a continuous monitoring technique in the neonatal intensive care unit. *Crit Care Med* 1988;16:1147–53.

32. Blaymore-Bier J, Pezzullo J, Kim E, Oh W, Garcia-Coll C, and Vohr BR. Outcome of extremely low-birth-weight infants: 1980–1990. *Acta Paediatr* December 1994;83(12):1244–48.

33. Saigal S, Rosenbaum P, Hattersley B, and Milner R. Decreased disability rate among 3-year-old survivors weighing 501 to 1000 grams at birth and born to residents of a geographically defined region from 1981 to 1984 compared with 1977 to 1980. *J Pediatr* 1989;114: 839–46.

34. Hack M, and Fanaroff AA. Outcomes of extremely-low-birth-weight infants between 1982 and 1988. *N Engl J Med* 1989;14;321:1642–47.

35. Roizen NJ, and Patterson D. Down's syndrome. *Lancet* 2003;361(9365):1281–89.

36. Leonard S, Bower C, Petterson B, and Leonard H. Survival of infants born with Down's syndrome: 1980–96. *Paediatr Perinat Epidemiol* 2000;14:163–71.

37. Pless JE. The story of baby doe. *N Engl J Med* 1983;309:664.

38. Meisel A. *The Right to Die.* New York: John Wiley and Sons, 1989:436–37.

39. Reagan R. *Abortion and the Conscience of the Nation.* New York: New Regency Publications, 2001.

40. Ibid.

41. Jennison J. Quoted in *US News and World Report,* January 16, 1984:63.

42. Babies and Big Brother. *Wall Street Journal,* February 28, 1984. Review and Outlook.

43. Big Brother in the nursery. *The Economist,* July 14, 1984:42.

44. Baby Doe needs no Big Brother. *New York Times,* July 26, 1983:A20.

45. Hentoff N. The awful privacy of Baby Doe. *The Atlantic,* January 1985:54.

46. Cited in Annas GJ. Checkmating the Baby Doe regulations. *Hastings Cent Rep* 1986; 14(4):29–31.

47. *Bown v. American Hospital Association,* 54 LW 4579 (June 9, 1986).

48. Department of Health and Human Services. Child abuse and neglect prevention and treatment programs. *Fed Regist* 1985;50:14878–901.

49. Koppelman LM, Irons TG, and Koppelman AE. Neonatologists judge the "Baby Doe" regulations. *N Engl J Med* 1988;318:677–83.

50. Haywood JL, Goldenberg RL, Bronstein J, Nelson KG, and Carlo WA. Comparison of perceived and actual rates of survival and freedom from handicap in premature infants. *Am J Obstet Gynecol* 1994;171:432–39.

51. Lee SK, Penner PL, and Cox M. Comparison of the attitudes of health care professionals and parents toward active treatment of very low birth weight infants. *Pediatrics* 1991; 88:110–14.

52. Hippocrates. The art. In Jones WH, ed. *Hippocrates II.* Cambridge, MA: Harvard, 1923:193.

53. Blackhall LJ. Must we always use CPR? *N Engl J Med* 1987;317:1281–85.

54. For some recent reviews of this literature, see Cantor MD, Braddock CH III, Derse AR, Edwards DM, Logue GL, Nelson W, Prudhomme AM, Pearlman RA, Reagan JE, Wlody

GS, Fox E; Veterans Health Administration National Ethics Committee. Do-not-resuscitate orders and medical futility. *Arch Intern Med* 2003;163:2689–94. Way J, Back AL, and Curtis JR. Withdrawing life support and resolution of conflict with families. *Br Med J* 2002;325(7376): 1342–45. Helft PR, Siegler M, and Lantos J. The rise and fall of the futility movement. *N Engl J Med* 2000;343:293–96.

55. Rhoden NK. Treating Baby Doe: The ethics of uncertainty. *Hastings Cent Rep* 1986; 15(4):34–42.

56. Ibid.

57. Lyon J. *Playing God in the Nursery.* New York: WW Norton, 1985:123–24.

58. Rothwell PM, McDowell Z, Wong CK, and Dorman PJ. Doctors and patients don't agree: cross sectional study of patients' and doctors' perceptions and assessments of disability in multiple sclerosis. *Br Med J* 1997;314(7094):1580–83.

59. Saigal S, Lambert M, Russ C, and Hoult L. Self-esteem of adolescents who were born prematurely. *Pediatrics* 2002;109:429–33. Feingold E, Sheir-Neiss G, Melnychuk J, Bachrach S, and Paul D. HRQL and severity of brain ultrasound findings in a cohort of adolescents who were born preterm. *J Adolesc Health* 2002;31(3):234–39.

60. Saigal S, Rosenbaum PL, Feeny D, Burrows E, Furlong W, Stoskopf BL, and Hoult L. Parental perspectives of the health status and health-related quality of life of teen-aged children who were extremely low birth weight and term controls. *Pediatrics* 2000;105: 569–74.

61. Siperstein GN, Wolraich ML, Reed D, and O'Keefe P. Medical decisions and prognostications of pediatricians for infants with meningomyelocele. *J Pediatr* 1988;113:835–40.

62. Streiner DL, Saigal S, Burrows E, Stoskopf B, and Rosenbaum P. Attitudes of parents and health care professionals toward active treatment of extremely premature infants. *Pediatrics* 2001;108:152–57.

63. Rhoden NK. Treatment dilemmas for imperiled newborns: why quality of life counts. *S Calif Law Rev* 1985;58:1283–1347.

64. NICHD Neonatal Research Network. Background and overview. Available at: http://neonatal.rti.org/about/network.cfm. Accessed October 14, 2005.

65. Vermont Oxford Network. Available at: www.vtoxford.org/. Accessed October 14, 2005.

66. Hack M, Horbar JD, Malloy MH, Tyson JE, Wright E, and Wright L. Very low birth weight outcomes of the National Institute of Child Health and Human Development Neonatal Network. *Pediatrics* 1991;87:587–97.

CHAPTER 5: THE END OF MEDICAL PROGRESS, 1992 TO PRESENT

1. Horbar JD, Badger GJ, Carpenter JH, Fanaroff AA, Kilpatrick S, LaCorte M, Phibbs R, and Soll RF. Trends in mortality and morbidity for very low birth weight infants, 1991–1999. *Pediatrics* 2002;110:143–51.

2. Hein HA, and Lofgren MA. The changing pattern of neonatal mortality in a regionalized system of perinatal care: A current update. *Pediatrics* 1999;104:1064–69.

3. Philip AG. Neonatal mortality rate: is further improvement possible? *J Pediatr* 1995; 126:427–33.

4. NIH Consensus Development Panel on the Effect of Corticosteroids for Fetal Maturation on Perinatal Outcomes. Effect of corticosteroids for feral maturation on perinatal outcomes. *JAMA* 1995;273:413–18.

5. Meadow W, Reimshisel T, and Lantos J. Birth weight-specific mortality for extremely low birth weight infants vanishes by four days of life: epidemiology and ethics in the neonatal intensive care unit. *Pediatrics* 1996;97(5):636–43.

6. Ellington M Jr, Richardson DK, Gray JE, and Pursley DM. Early deaths in Chicago and New England. *Pediatrics* 1997;99:753–54.

7. Richardson DK, Gray JE, McCormick MC, Workman K, and Goldmann DA. Score for neonatal acute physiology: a physiologic severity index for neonatal intensive care. *Pediatrics* 1993;91(3):617–23.

8. Meadow W, Frain L, Ren Y, Lee G, Soneji S, and Lantos J. Serial assessment of mortality in the neonatal intensive care unit by algorithm and intuition: certainty, uncertainty, and informed consent. *Pediatrics* 2002;109(5):878–86.

9. Ibid.

10. Wood NS, Marlow N, Costeloe K, Gibson AT, and Wilkinson AR. Neurologic and developmental disability after extremely preterm birth. EPICure Study Group. *N Engl J Med* 2000;343:378–84.

11. D'Angio CT, Sinkin RA, Stevens TP, Landfish NK, Merzbach JL, Ryan RNM, Phelps DL, Palumbo DR, and Myers GS. Longitudinal, fifteen-year follow-up of children born at less than 29 weeks' gestation after introduction of surfactant therapy into a region: neurologic, cognitive, and educational outcomes. *Pediatrics* 2002;110(6):1094–102.

12. Vohr BR, Wright LL, Dusick AM, Mele L, Verter J, Steichen JJ, Simon NP, Wilson DC, Broyles S, Bauer CR, et al. Neurodevelopmental and functional outcomes of extremely low birth weight infants in the National Institute of Child Health and Human Development Neonatal Research Network, 1993–1994. *Pediatrics* 2000;105:1216–26.

13. *Miller v. HCA*, 47 Tex Sup J 12, 118 SW3d 758 (2003).

14. This case summary is available on a Michigan State University Web site. Children and infants—case for discussion: the Messenger case. Available at: www.msu.edu/course/hm/546/messenger.htm.

15. *Montalvo v. Borkovek-Montalvo*, 2002 WI App 147.

16. Ibid.

17. Ibid.

18. Kostelanetz AS, and Dhanireddy R. Survival of the very-low-birth-weight infants after cardiopulmonary resuscitation in neonatal intensive care unit. *J Perinatol* 2004;24:279–83.

19. Larroque B, Breart G, Kaminski M, Dehan M, Andre M, Burguet A, Grandjean H, Ledesert B, Leveque C, Maillard F, et al.; Epipage study group. Survival of very preterm infants: Epipage, a population based cohort study. *Arch Dis Child Fetal Neonatal Ed* 2004;89:F139–44.

20. Annas GJ. Asking the courts to set the standard of emergency care—the case of Baby K. *N Engl J Med* 1994;330:1542–45.

21. Roizen NJ, and Patterson D. Down's syndrome. *Lancet* 2003;361(9365):1281–89.

22. Forrester MB, and Merz RD. First-year mortality rates for selected birth defects, Hawaii, 1986–1999. *Am J Med Genet* 2003;119A(3):311–18.

23. Society of Critical Care Medicine Ethics Committee. Attitudes of critical care medicine professionals concerning forgoing life-sustaining treatments. *Crit Care Med* 1992;20: 320–26.

24. Asch DA, Faber-Langendoen K, Shea JA, and Christakis NA. The sequence of withdrawing life-sustaining treatment from patients. *Am J Med* 1999;107:153–56.

25. Truog RD. "Doctor, if this were your child, what would you do"? *Pediatrics* 1999; 103:153–54.

26. Sacks O. *A Leg to Stand On*. New York: Touchstone, 1998.

27. Murphy RF. *The Body Silent*. New York: WW Norton, 1990:24–25.

28. Meyers C. Cruel choices: autonomy and critical care decision-making. *Bioethics* 2004;18:104–19.

29. Dostoevsky F. *The Brothers Karamazov*. trans. Garnett C. New York: Signet, 1957:251–52.

30. Lantos J, Robins Z, and Meadow W. Negotiating neonatal deaths—bioethical dreams and emotional realities. *Pediatr Res* 1999;45:347.

31. Oe K. *A Personal Matter*. trans. Nathan J. New York: Grove, 1969:74–76.

32. Garros D, Rosychuk RJ, and Cox PN. Circumstances surrounding end of life in a pediatric intensive care unit. *Pediatrics* 2003;112(5):e371. Meyer EC, Burns JP, Griffith JL, and Truog RD. Parental perspectives on end-of-life care in the pediatric intensive care unit. *Crit Care Med* 2002;30:226–31.

33. Wall SN, and Partridge JC. Death in the intensive care nursery: physician practice of withdrawing and withholding life support. *Pediatrics* 1997;99:64–70.

34. Singh J, Lantos J, and Meadow W. End-of-life after birth: death and dying in a neonatal intensive care unit. *Pediatrics* 2004;114:1620–26.

CHAPTER 6: ECONOMICS OF THE NICU

1. Rogowski J. Measuring the cost of neonatal and perinatal care. *Pediatrics* 1999;103: 329–35.

2. Strunk BC, and Ginsburg PB. Trends: Tracking health care costs: trends turn downward in 2003. *Health Aff* (Millwood) June 2004;W4.

3. Lewit EM, Baker LS, Corman H, Shiono PH. The direct cost of low birth weight. *Future Child* 1995;5:35–56.

4. Ibid.

5. Levit KR, Lazenby HC, and Sivarajan L. Health care spending in 1994: slowest in decades. *Health Aff* (Millwood) 1996;15(2):130–44.

6. Cowan C, Catlin A, Smith C, and Sensenig A. National health expenditures, 2002. *Health Care Financ Rev* 2004;25(4):143–66.

7. Boyle MH, Torrance GW, Sinclair JC, and Horwood SP. Economic evaluation of neonatal intensive care of very-low-birth-weight infants. *N Engl J Med* 1983;308:1330–37.

8. Stolz JW, and McCormick MC. Restricting access to neonatal intensive care: effect on mortality and economic savings. *Pediatrics* March 1998;101(3 pt 1):344–48.

9. Doyle LW; Victorian Infant Collaborative Study Group. Evaluation of neonatal intensive care for extremely low birth weight infants in Victoria over two decades: II. Efficiency. *Pediatrics* March 2004;113(3 pt 1):510–14.

10. Merkens MJ, and Garland MJ. The Oregon Health Plan and the ethics of care for marginally viable newborns. *J Clin Ethics* Fall 2001;12(3):266–74. Jakobi P, Weissman A, and Paldi E. The extremely low birthweight infant: the twenty-first century dilemma. *Am J Perinatol* 1993;10(2):155–59.

11. Roberton NR. Should we look after babies less than 800 g? *Arch Dis Child* 1993;68 (3 Spec No):326–29.

12. Eriksson M, and Lindroth M. Ethical dilemmas in Swedish neonatal intensive care. *J Clin Ethics* 2001;12:312–14.

13. Yu VY, Bajuk B, and Hollingsworth E. Neonatal intensive care for extremely low birthweight infants: a dilemma in perinatal medicine. *Aust Paediatr J* December 1981; 262–64.

14. Lantos JD, Mokalla M, and Meadow W. Resource allocation in neonatal and medical ICUs. Epidemiology and rationing at the extremes of life. *Am J Respir Crit Care Med* 1997; 156:185–89.

15. Hack M, and Fanaroff AA. Outcomes of extremely-low-birth-weight infants between 1982 and 1988. *N Engl J Med* 1989;321:1642–47.

16. Ellington M Jr, Richardson DK, Gray JE, and Pursley DM. Early deaths in Chicago and New England. *Pediatrics* 1997;99:753–54.

17. Meadow W, Lee G, Lin K, and Lantos J. Changes in mortality for extremely low birth weight infants in the 1990s: implications for treatment decisions and resource use. *Pediatrics* 2004;113:1223–29.

18. Gustaitis R, and Young E. *A Time to Be Born, A Time to Die: Conflicts and Ethics in an Intensive Care Nursery*. Boston: Pearson Addison Wesley, 1986:212.

19. U.S. Department of Health and Human Services. *Health United States, 1995*. DHHS Publication Number (PHS) 96-1232. Hyattsville, Md. May 1996:203.

20. Hughes DM, McLeod M, Garner B, and Goldbloom RB. Controlled trial of a home and ambulatory program for asthmatic children. *Pediatrics* 1991;87:54–61. Morray B, and Redding G. Factors associated with prolonged hospitalization of children with asthma. *Arch Pediatr Adolesc Med* 1995;149:276–79.

21. Hirasing RA, Reeser HM, de Groot RR, Ruwaard D, van Buren S, and Verloove-Vanhorick SP. Trends in hospital admissions among children aged 0–19 years with type I diabetes in The Netherlands. *Diabetes Care* 1996;19:431–34.

22. Pestian JP, Derkay CS, and Ritter C. Outpatient tonsillectomy and adenoidectomy clinical pathways: an evaluative study. *Am J Otolaryngol* 1998;19:45–49.

23. Saenz NC, Conlon KC, Aronson DC, and LaQuaglia MP. The application of minimal access procedures in infants, children, and young adults with pediatric malignancies. *J Laparoendosc Adv Surg Tech* 1997;7:289–94.

24. Wacker P, Halperin DS, Wyss M, and Humbert J. Early hospital discharge of children with fever and neutropenia: a prospective study. *J Pediatr Hematol Oncol* 1997;19:208–11.

25. Lantos JD. Hooked on neonatology. *Health Aff* (Millwood) 2001;20(5):233–40.

26. South Shore hospital bond rating downgraded. *Boston Business Journal*. August 30, 2002. Available at: www.bizjournals.com/boston/stories/2002/08/26/daily58.html. Accessed October 14, 2005.

27. S. Shore hospital will build NICU. *Boston Business Journal*. November 21, 2002. Available at: www.bizjournals.com/boston/stories/2002/11/18/daily34.html. Accessed October 14, 2005.

28. Howell EM, Richardson D, Ginsburg P, and Foot B. Deregionalization of neonatal intensive care in urban areas. *Am J Public Health* January 2002;92(1):119–24.

29. Cifuentes J, Bronstein J, Phibbs CS, Phibbs RH, Schmitt SK, and Carlo WA. Mortality in low birth weight infants according to level of neonatal care at hospital of birth. *Pediatrics* 2002;109:745–51.

30. Meadow W, Kim M, Mendez D, Bell A, Gray C, Corpuz M, and Lantos J. Which nurseries currently care for ventilated neonates in Illinois and Wisconsin? Implications for the next generation of perinatal regionalization. *Am J Perinatol* 2002;19:197–203.

31. Thompson LA, Goodman DC, and Little GA. Is more neonatal intensive care always better? Insights from a cross-national comparison of reproductive care. *Pediatrics* 2002;109(6):1036–43.

32. Lorenz JM, Paneth N, Jetton JR, den Ouden L, and Tyson JE. Comparison of management strategies for extreme prematurity in New Jersey and the Netherlands: outcomes and resource expenditure. *Pediatrics* 2001;108:1269–74.

33. Lantos, Hooked on neonatology.

CHAPTER 7: FOUR DISCARDED MORAL CHOICES

1. Wegman ME. Annual summary of vital statistics, 1966. *Pediatrics* 1967;40:1035–45.

2. Chase HC. The position of the United States in international comparisons of health status. *Am J Public Health* 1972;62:581–89.

3. Sinclair JC, Torrance GW, Boyle MH, Horwood SP, Saigal S, and Sackett DL. Evaluation of neonatal-intensive-care programs. *N Engl J Med* 1981;305:489–94.

4. Silverman WA. Neonatal pediatrics at the century mark. *Perspect Biol Med* 1989;32:159–69.

5. Kliegman RM. Neonatal technology, perinatal survival, social consequences, and the perinatal paradox. *Am J Public Health* July 1995;85(7):909–13.

6. Institute of Medicine, Committee to Study the Prevention of Low Birthweight. *Preventing Low Birthweight*. Washington, D.C.: National Academy Press, 1985:233.

7. U.S. Congress, Office of Technology Assessment. *Health Children: Investing in the Future*. Washington, D.C.: U.S. Government Printing Office, 1988.

8. Quoted in Sardell A. Child health policy in the US. The paradox of consensus. *J Health Polit Policy Law* 1990;15:271–304.

9. Huntington J, and Connell FA. For every dollar spent: the cost-savings argument for prenatal care. *N Engl J Med* 1994;331:1303–7.

10. Becker ER, and Teutsch SM. State maternal and child expenditures and low birth-weight infants: a descriptive analysis. *J Health Care Finance* 2000;27(1):1–10.

11. Paneth N. Tiny babies, enormous costs. *Birth* 1992;19:154–61.

12. Hack M, and Fanaroff AA. Outcomes of extremely immature infants: a perinatal dilemma. *N Engl J Med* 1993;329:1649–50.

13. Hadorn DC. The problem of discrimination in health care priority setting. *JAMA* 1992;268:1454–59.

14. Silverman WA. Overtreatment of neonates? A personal retrospective. *Pediatrics* December 1992;90(6):971–76.

15. Anderson P, and Doyle L. Neurobehavioral outcomes of school-age children born extremely low birth weight or very preterm in the 1990s. *JAMA* 2003;289:3264–72.

16. Saigal S, den Ouden L, Wolke D, Hoult L, Paneth N, Streiner DL, Whitaker A, and Pinto-Martin J. School-age outcomes in children who were extremely low birth weight from four international population-based cohorts. *Pediatrics* 2003;112:943–50.

17. Wichers MJ, van der Schouw YT, Moons KG, Stam HJ, and van Nieuwenhuizen O. Prevalence of cerebral palsy in The Netherlands (1977–1988). *Eur J Epidemiol* 2001;17(6):527–32.

18. Pharoah PO, Platt MJ, and Cooke T. The changing epidemiology of cerebral palsy. *Arch Dis Child Fetal Neonatal Ed* 1996;75:F169–73.

19. Clark FA. Reported rates of cerebral palsy, 1966–1996. *Am J Obstet Gynecol* 2003;188: 628–33.

20. Lorenz JM, Wooliever DE, Jetton JR, and Paneth N. A quantitative review of mortality and developmental disability in extremely premature newborns. *Arch Pediatr Adolesc Med* 1998;152:425–35.

21. Winter S, Autry A, Boyle C, and Yeargin-Allsopp M. Trends in the prevalence of cerebral palsy in a population-based study. *Pediatrics* 2002;110:1220–25.

22. Silverman WA. Restraining the unsustainable. *Pediatrics* 2003;111:672–74.

23. Paris JJ, Schrieber MD, and Reardon F. The "emergent circumstances" exception to the need for consent: The Texas Supreme Court ruling in Miller v. HCA. *J Perinatol* 2004; 24:337–42.

24. American Academy of Pediatrics Committee on Fetus and Newborn, American College of Obstetrics and Gynecologists Committee on Obstetric Practice. Perinatal care at the threshold of viability. *Pediatrics* 1995;96:974–76.

25. Paris JJ, and Schreiber MD. Physicians' refusal to provide life-prolonging medical interventions. *Clin Perinatol* 1996;23:563–71.

26. Koop CE. The slide to Auschwitz. The Pro-Life Forum. Accessed at http://www.prolifeforum.org/ethics/everett.asp on July 14, 2004.

27. McCormick RA. The quality of life, the sanctity of life. *Hastings Cent Rep* February 1978;30–66.

CHAPTER 8: THE POSSIBILITY OF MORAL PROGRESS

1. President's Council on Bioethics. Human cloning and human dignity: an ethical inquiry. Available at: www.bioethics.gov/reports/cloningreport/recommend.html. Accessed October 14, 2005.

Index

abortion, U.S. Supreme Court and, 68, 69, 72

American Academy of Family Physicians (AAFP), 43

American Academy of Pediatrics (AAP), 43, 65, 74

American Coalition of Citizens with Disabilities, 71

American College of Obstetrics and Gynecology (ACOG), 43, 65

American Medical Association (AMA), Committee on Maternal and Child Care, 43

anencephaly, 110, 111

Annas, George, 5

antenatal steroids, 62–64

Association for Retarded Citizens, 71

Association for the Severely Handicapped, 71

Baby Doe controversy: Child Abuse and Treatment Act and, 73–74; effects of, 74–83; legal facts of, 67–68; medical facts of, 66–67; social and political ramifications of, 68–72; U.S. Supreme Court and, 72–73

Bartlett, R. H., 57, 58

Becker, E. R., 141

birthweight: life-sustaining treatment and, 90, 92; outcome and, 98–99, 143–146; predictive power of, 85–90, 92, 109; programs to prevent low, 140–142; rationing based on, 126–127. See also extremely low birthweight (ELBW) infants; very low birthweight (VLBW) infants

Bradley, Bill, 140

The Brothers Karamazov (Dostoevsky), 115–117

Burks, Shemika A., 107

Burks v. St. Joseph Hospital, 107

Butterfield, L. Joseph, 43

California, regionalization in, 46

Campbell, Arthur, 47–49

Castle, Michael N., 140

cerebral palsy (CP), 143–146

Chain, Ernst, 19

Child Abuse and Treatment Act (CAPTA) of 1984: amendments to, 73–76; withholding treatment and, 107

child abuse/neglect, 50–51, 82–83

children: born ELBW, 144; inpatient stays for, 130, 131

Chiles, Lawton, 140

Chu, J., 54

clinical intuition, 95–96, 99

clinical practice, 22, 28

clinical research: acquisition of knowledge in, 28–29; line between clinical practice and, 22, 28; trials in, 25–27

Coghill, Robert, 19

cognitive deficits: long-term outcome and, 96, 97; quality of life and, 79–80

Committee on Maternal and Child Care (American Medical Association), 43

Committee on Perinatal Health Report (1976), 43

communication, neonatal decision making and, 104–106, 113, 119

congenital abnormalities: explanation of, 14; treatment of infants with, 15

continuous positive airway pressure (CPAP): long-term follow-up of, 32–33; research on, 31–32

Costellano, Carol, 4
Crowley, P., 63

decision making: "broad shoulders" approach
    to, 114–115; consensus about process and,
    119–121; nature of medical, 113–115; objective
    information approach to, 113–114; prenatal,
    101–105, 108; shared deniability approach to,
    115–119. *See also* neonatal decision making
Delivoria-Papadopoulos, M., 24, 25, 59
Disabilities Rights Education and Defense
    Fund, 71
do not resuscitate orders, 108
Down syndrome: Baby Doe and, 66–67;
    obligatory treatment for, 110, 111; parental
    treatment decisions and, 49
Dudrick, S. J., 33, 34
Duff, Raymond, 47, 48

economic issues: ethics and, 125–126, 129, 135;
    NICU cost-effectiveness and, 125–129; NICUs
    and hospital finance and, 129–131; NICUs as
    profit centers and, 6, 130; overall costs of
    NICU care and, 123–125; overview of,
    122–123; perinatal regionalization and, 44,
    132–135
Elbourne, D., 59–60
Elder, Albert, 19
eligibility criteria: decisions regarding, 25–27;
    explanation of, 30
Ellis, T. S., 50, 51
epidermolysis bullosa, 80–81
ethics: analysis of, 36–40; economics and,
    125–126, 129, 135; guidelines for, 40–41;
    historical background of, 9–10; present
    consensus and, 136–138; science vs., 150–151;
    toward progress in, 151–154. *See also* moral
    views
euthanasia, passive vs. active, 39
exogenous surfactant therapy, 55
extracorporeal membrane oxygenation
    (ECMO): development of, 57–58; evaluation
    process for, 54, 59; use of, 58–60
extremely low birthweight (ELBW) infants:
    clinical intuition study and, 95–96, 99; follow-
    up program for, 83; long-term outcomes of,
144; outcome and, 98, 99; quality of life issues
    and, 78. *See also* very low birthweight
    (VLBW) infants

financial issues. *See* economic issues
Fleming, Alexander, 18, 19
Fletcher, Joseph, 39, 40, 49
Florey, Howard, 19
Food and Drug Administration (FDA), 56, 57
"For Every Dollar Spent—The Cost Savings
    Argument for Prenatal Care" (Huntington
    and Connell), 141
Fost, N., 49
Frey, Darcy, 5
Fujiwara, T., 55, 56
full-term infants, 14–15

group B streptococcal (GBS): in infants, 64–65;
    screening of pregnant women for, 62, 64–65
Gustafson, James, 49
Gustaitis, R., 130

Heatley, Norman, 19
Hentoff, Nat, 71
Hess, Julius, 23
high-frequency oscillating ventilation (HFOV), 54
Hippocrates, 76
Horbar, J. D., 55, 59
Hospital Corporation of America, 100
hospitals: economics of NICUs and, 129–131;
    regional neonatal program development and,
    44–47; trends in NICU, 132
Howie R. N., 63
Hyde, Henry J., 140
hypothesis testing, 29

idiopathic respiratory distress syndrome (IRDS),
    continuous positive airway pressure to treat,
    31–32
Illinois, regionalization in, 44–45
illness, 114
infant mortality: explanation of, 13; trends in,
    13–14, 17. *See also* neonatal mortality
informed consent, 106–107
innovation. *See* medical innovation
Institute of Medicine (IOM), 140

intermittent positive pressure respiration (IPPR): eligibility criteria for, 25–26, 28, 29; ethical issues and, 29–31; implications of research findings and, 30–31; initial research on, 24, 25, 35; nature of research on, 29–30; techniques and methodologies for, 27–28

Jacobs, Marc, 100–101

Kennedy, John F., 139
Kliegman, R. M., 140
Koop, C. Everett, 148
Kwong, M. S., 55

Lee, S. K., 75
legal issues: nature of law and, 107–108; prenatal decision making and, 101–105, 108; on withholding/withdrawing treatment, 47–49, 100–108
Leland, Mickey, 140
Levison, H., 24
Liggins, G. C., 63
long-term outcomes, 96–99
Lorenz, M. J., 145
Lucey, Jerold, 37

Madden, Jack, 45
malpractice cases, 100. *See also* legal issues
March of Dimes, 43
Massachusetts, regionalization in, 46
McCormick, Richard, 149
McDonald v. Milleville, 105–106
mechanical ventilation: clinical trials for, 25–27; development of, 23–33, 53; successful use of, 33
Medicaid, 123, 129–130, 140
medical futility, 76–77
medical innovation: examples of, 18–20; mechanical ventilation as, 23–33; in neonatology, 3–4, 20–23; total parenteral nutrition as, 33–36
Medicare, 123
Meisel, A., 67
Messinger, Gregory, 103–105
Meyers, C., 114
Miller, Carla, 100–102
Miller v. HCA, 100–102, 107, 147

Montalvo, Nancy, 106
moral views: harm to survivors and, 143–146; parental decision making and, 146–148; present consensus and, 136–138; preventive care and, 138–143; sanctity of life vs. quality of life and, 148–149. *See also* ethics
mortality. *See* neonatal mortality

National Institute of Child Health and Development Neonatal Research Network, 83
near-term infants, 14–15
neonatal decision making: clinical facts and, 108–111; communication and, 104–106, 113, 119; consensus about process and, 119–121; elements of, 4–5; moral psychology of, 111–119; parental, 48–49, 52, 100; prognostication and, 88–90; societal oversight of, 99–100; at time of birth, 101–109. *See also* decision making
neonatal intensive care: effects of, 139, 143–146; efficiency of, 127; funding in Europe for, 134–135; legal cases in 1970s and, 47–52; mechanical ventilation and, 23–33, 35, 36, 53; moral issues in 1960s and 1970s in, 36–41; progress in, 154–156; randomized controlled trials and, 60–62; regionalization and, 41–47; total parenteral nutrition and, 33–36, 53
neonatal intensive care units (NICUs): cost-effectiveness of, 125–129; economic issues and, 6, 44; financial issues and, 6, 44; full-term or near-term infants in, 14–15; hospital finance and, 129–131; infants with congenital anomalies in, 14, 15; infants with extreme prematurity in, 14–16; inpatient days in, 130–131; overall costs of, 123–125; power structure in, 113; practice refinements in 1980s in, 65–66; realities of, 5–6; treatment decisions and, 4–5
neonatal mortality: birthweight-specific, 85–92, 133; causes of, 23; explanation of, 13; time to death and, 127, 128; trends in, 14, 133, 138–139
Neonatal Research Network (National Institute of Child Health and Development), 83
neonatologists: Baby Doe regulations and, 74–75; prediction of outcomes of premature infants by, 75–76, 88; statistics for, 134. *See also* pediatricians

neonatology: historical background of, 8–10; leveling off of progress in, 85–88; medical innovation in, 3–4, 20–23, 85; moral ambiguities in, 4–8; overview of, 1–3

neurological deficits: long-term outcome and, 96, 97; neonatal intensive care and, 143–146

obstetricians, 75

Osler, William, 19

Otero, Eduardo, 101, 102

oxygenation, 21

Paneth, N., 143

parents: consensus decisions with, 119–121; empowerment of, 113; malpractice cases initiated by, 100–102; treatment decisions and, 48–49, 52, 100–108, 112–114, 146–148; views on withholding vs. withdrawing treatment, 112

Parents of Blind Children–New Jersey, 4

Paris, John, 4–5, 146–148

pediatricians, 75–79, 88. *See also* neonatologists

penicillin, 18–20

perinatal regionalization: development of, 41–47; economics of, 132–135; goals of, 47

A Personal Matter (Oe), 118

Pettigrew, Ann, 46

positive-pressure ventilation: development of, 23–24; effects of long-term, 31

postneonatal mortality, 13

premature infants: causes of death in, 23; predicting outcome of, 75, 77, 109; respiratory distress in, 23; treatment of, 15–17. *See also* birthweight; extremely low birthweight (ELBW) infants; very low birthweight (VLBW) infants

prenatal care, 140–142

prenatal decision making, 101–105, 108. *See also* decision making; neonatal decision making

President's Commission on Bioethics Report (1982), 90, 146

President's Council on Bioethics (2005), 156

"Prevention Low Birthweight" (Institute of Medicine), 140

preventive care: moral issues and, 138–143; screening of pregnant women for group B streptococcal colonization as, 62, 64–65; steroid therapy for women in premature labor as, 62–64

prognostication: clinical intuition and, 95–96, 99; ethical decision making and, 88–90; long-term, 88, 96–99; pediatrician, 75–79, 88; refinements to, 90–96; short-term, 88; SNAP score and, 92–95

quality of life: assumptions regarding, 78; components of, 79–81; decision making and, 110–111; sanctity of life vs., 148–149

Quinlan, Karen, 51

Rachels, James, 39

Raju, T. N., 55

Randolph, Judson, 40

randomized controlled trials (RCTs), 60–62

Reagan, Ronald, 69–71

regionalization. *See* perinatal regionalization

Rehabilitation Act of 1973, 68, 70, 72, 73

respiratory distress: advances in treatment of, 23; approaches to treatment of, 31–33; CMO and, 57–61; surfactant and, 54–57

Rhoden, Nancy, 77

Robertson, J. A., 49

Roe v. Wade, 68, 69, 72

Saigal, S., 78, 144

sanctity of life, 148–149

severe respiratory distress syndrome, 24

Shapiro, D. L., 55

Shaw, Anthony, 48, 49

short gut syndrome, 81

Silverman, W. A., 20, 21, 139, 146–147

Siperstein, G. N., 78–79

SNAP scores: explanation of, 92–93; limitations of, 93–95

South Shore Hospital, 131

Stahlman, Mildred, 38

state health departments, 45–46

Supreme Court, U.S.: abortion and, 68, 69; Baby Doe regulations and, 72–73

surfactant: development of, 54–56, 87; testing of, 56–57, 59

Swyer, P. R., 24

Teutsch, S. M., 141
Thompson, L. A., 134
total parenteral nutrition (TPN), 33–36, 53
tracheal intubation, 25
trial of therapy: birthweight and, 92, 99;
    time-limited nature of, 108
Trisomy 13, 111
Trisomy 18, 110–111
Truog, R. D., 113

University of Chicago Hospitals (UCHs):
    financial information for, 131; NICU data
    from, 86–87; regionalized NICUs and, 44–45

Veatch, Robert, 39–40
Vermont-Oxford Consortium, 83–85

very low birthweight (VLBW) infants: costs
    and length of stay for, 124; mortality rates
    and, 87; predicting outcome for, 75;
    regionalization and, 47. See also extremely
    low birthweight (ELBW) infants
Vila, Brian, 106

Waxman, Henry, 140
Whittier, Gayle, 5
Wichers, M. J., 144–145
withdrawing treatment, 112
withholding treatment, 112

Yale–New Haven Hospital, 47–48
Young, E., 130

ABOUT THE AUTHORS

John D. Lantos, M.D., is professor of pediatrics and medicine, chief of the Section of General Pediatrics, and associate director of the MacLean Center for Clinical Medical Ethics at the University of Chicago. He has a B.A. in semiotics from Brown University and an M.D. from the University of Pittsburgh. His previous books include *Do We Still Need Doctors?* (Routledge, 1997) and *The Lazarus Case* (Johns Hopkins, 2001). He is co-editor of *Primum Non Nocere Today* (Elsevier, 1995) and *The Last Physician: Walker Percy and the Moral Life of Medicine* (Duke, 1999).

William L. Meadow, M.D., Ph.D., is professor of pediatrics and medicine and co-chief of the Section of Neonatology at the University of Chicago, where he has been on the faculty since 1981. He received his M.D. and Ph.D. (in physiology) from the University of Pennsylvania. Dr. Meadow has published extensively in the field of neonatal septic shock. More recently, he has turned to studying the interaction between clinical epidemiology and ethical decision making in the neonatal ICU.